Wound Healing: A systematic approach to advanced wound healing and management

Other titles available from Wounds UK include:

Honey: A modern wound management product
edited by Richard White, Rose Cooper and Peter Molan

Essential Wound Management: An introduction for undergraduates
by David Gray, John Timmons and Pam Cooper

A Pocket Guide to Clinical Decision-making in Wound Management
edited by David Gray and Sue Bale

Skin Care in Wound Management: Assessment, prevention and treatment
edited by Richard White

Wounds UK — The Directory, 2006 edited by Richard White
and Clare Morris

Wound Healing: A systematic approach to advanced wound healing and management

edited by

David Gray and Pam Cooper

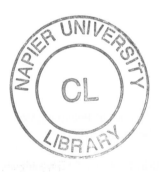

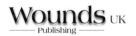

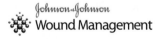

Wounds UK Publishing, Wounds UK Limited, Suite 3.1, 36 Upperkirkgate, Aberdeen AB10 1BA

British Library Cataloguing-in-Publication Data
A catalogue record is available for this book

ISBN 0-9549193-5-1

Printed in the UK by Cromwell Press, Trowbridge, Wiltshire

CONTENTS

List of contributors   vii

Foreword by Andrew Kingsley   ix

Introduction by David Gray   xi

Chapter 1   Assessment of a patient with a wound   1
              Eva-Lisa Heinrichs, Mair Llewellyn and Keith Harding

Chapter 2   A review of different wound types and their   28
              principles of management
              Pam Cooper

Chapter 3   Applied Wound Management   59
              David Gray, Richard White, Pam Cooper
              and Andrew Kingsley

Chapter 4   Case studies   101
              Pam Cooper

Appendix   Applied Wound Management tools   113
              David Gray

Index   121

LIST OF CONTRIBUTORS

Pam Cooper is a Clinical Nurse Specialist in Tissue Viability, Grampian NHS Acute Trust, Aberdeen.

David Gray is a Clinical Nurse Specialist in Tissue Viability, Grampian NHS Acute Trust, Aberdeen.

Keith Harding is Director of the Wound Healing Research Unit, Professor of Rehabilitation Medicine (wound healing), Cardiff University, Cardiff.

Eva-Lisa Heinrichs is Clinical Research Fellow, Wound Healing Research Unit, Cardiff University, Cardiff.

Andrew Kingsley is Tissue Viability Nurse Specialist, North Devon District Hospital, Barnstaple.

Mair Llewellyn is Patient Services Facilitator, Wound Healing Research Unit, Cardiff University, Cardiff.

Richard White is Senior Research Fellow, Department of Tissue Viability, Aberdeen Royal Infirmary, Aberdeen.

FOREWORD

One of the great challenges in wound management is consistency of approach between different professionals in a team, and between teams at national and international levels. There are many obstacles to achieving this, including problems with the evidence base for specific interventions, varying local formularies and funding, clinician preferences and training, and the absence of common documentation. In recent years, the welcome arrival of the concept of Wound Bed Preparation has focused our minds on the underlying pathophysiology of chronic wounds, encouraging clinicians to employ treatment aimed at the particular issues that these wounds present. This concept has currently been developed into the tabular guide known as TIME, and provides a quick reference to the mechanisms underlying the problem wound, and potential interventions with which to address the barriers to healing. However, there remains a need in clinical practice to provide a system for assessing the wound, and monitoring the outcomes of the interventions taken, in a simple and quick manner, utilising the available cues provided by the wound.

Applied Wound Management (AWM) is an important and emerging system that does just that, providing a clear monitor of progress both good and bad, which is easily used by all members of the healthcare team. Using the system will enhance communication within teams, and between teams, as the patient moves through the healthcare system. AWM comes in paper and electronic formats, allowing teams with different record systems to adopt the concept. Looking into the future, as the development of the electronic patient record gathers pace in the UK, AWM is positioned to become a powerful national platform for wound management. If we all use the same system, communicating about our patients will become easier and be in their best interests. From the local service perspective, being able to demonstrate the cost and clinical advantages of good wound care will help to highlight the value of maintaining and developing this area of practice. At the national level, the gathering of epidemiological data will enhance the visibility of the problem of wounds and the need for robust services to provide the care.

This book supports the idea of the need for doctors to be involved in the diagnostic stage of wound management, arguing that their skills make them ideally placed to consider the wound in the wider context of the health of the patient. Getting sufficient medics interested and involved in a structured way remains a challenge. The doctors will come when we construct a robust national wound service with primary, secondary and tertiary referral points. However, before this can be achieved, we must adopt a single approach to wound assessment to prove our serious intent to work together in a systematic fashion, and do some counting to persuade 'the powers that be' that wounds are worth investing in for the good of the country at large. AWM has the potential to make the difference and I commend the system and this book to you: new century health care, needs new century solutions.

Andrew Kingsley
Tissue Viability Nurse Specialist
North Devon District Hospital
October, 2005

INTRODUCTION

Applied Wound Management is a method of wound assessment and documentation which seeks to facilitate clinical decision-making, communication between professionals, and clinical audit. This book is one of a number of tools which include, articles, journal supplements, clinical tools, clinical audit software, professional seminars and web-based resources, which aim to support the practitioner in the use of Applied Wound Management. Applied Wound Management is a Wounds UK initiative, developed in partnership with Johnson and Johnson Advanced Wound Management.

David Gray
Clinical Director
Wounds UK
October, 2005

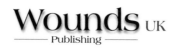
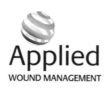
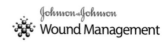

CHAPTER 1

ASSESSMENT OF A PATIENT WITH A WOUND

Eva-Lisa Heinrichs, Mair Llewellyn and Keith Harding

Introduction

In a healthy individual, wound healing usually proceeds in a predictable sequential manner, and the involvement of a specialised healthcare professional is seldom required. Nevertheless, difficulties arise when wound healing does not progress according to plan. There are several guidelines for the assessment and management of wounds; however, they tend to be based on specific wound types, where the origin and type of the wound have already been diagnosed or assumed. It has also been stated that without careful attention to pressure reduction, infection, necrotic tissue, tissue perfusion, nutrition, mobility, pain and psychosocial issues, as a total package, wounds will not heal. While this is certainly true, the initial key to a successful outcome for the patient is an accurate diagnosis of the underlying aetiology of the wound. An inadequate or incorrect diagnosis could prolong the duration of the wound, result in loss of time or limb, and/or further exacerbate the patient's condition, with associated increased morbidity and mortality, as well as greater cost to the patient and society.

A wound should always be assessed in the context of the patient's overall medical status and history, the presenting symptoms, and results of investigations, as well as the indicators for success or failure of treatment. Focusing on the 'whole patient and not just the hole in the patient' is essential to ensure that the underlying aetiology of the wound is known, and to ensure that the subsequent treatment plan is optimal for each patient.

Over the years, many physicians have been frustrated by their inability to help patients deal with their wounds. With rising medical costs, and increasing patient loads, physicians find themselves with less time to spend on an individual patient's ongoing care. It is also unnecessary in many cases for physicians to become involved in the day-to-day management and follow-up of patients with wounds. However, it is important that the physician, as a member of a multidisciplinary team caring for patients with wounds, has a role at the stage of making the initial diagnosis and, if necessary, in any subsequent modifications of the initial diagnosis. A physician is likely to be best placed among the members of the team by virtue of his/her specific training, knowledge and experience, to consider and to assess the various factors required for a correct diagnosis. The diagnosis and cause of a wound should be established as accurately and as early as possible, and appropriate treatment started quickly to avoid unnecessary suffering and increased risk to the patient. Only a thorough knowledge of possible underlying or related pathologies and other factors, such as patients' medication, will alert the examiner to explore further clues in the medical history, or clues in the overall patient examination which otherwise may be neglected or missed. If the patient is to receive optimal care from a multidisciplinary team, the physician should be involved in the taking of the patient's medical history, and in the examination of the patient as a whole.

As well as providing a review of some of the most common wound aetiologies, this chapter will highlight the importance of a holistic approach to the assessment and treatment of patients with wounds, offering suggestions for a structured approach to the diagnosis and management of wounds.

HEIDI — a tool in wound assessment and care

When examining a patient with a wound, a clinician is faced with several questions and decisions that require information-gathering before a diagnostic hypothesis can be made. To help practitioners make informed clinical decisions, and to have a structured approach to the assessment, diagnosis and management of any type of wound, a useful framework has been created, which focuses on the patient as a whole, rather than the hole in the patient. This framework is known by the acronym HEIDI. HEIDI stands for what we consider to be the five most important aspects of assessing and managing patients with wounds:

❖ **History** — relevant

- ❖ **Examination** — appropriate
- ❖ **Investigations** — necessary
- ❖ **Diagnosis** — likely or definite
- ❖ **Indicators** — of progress or complications

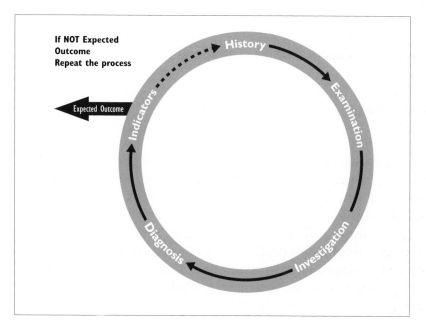

Figure 1.1: HEIDI: A framework for wound assessment

History

The treatment of all wounds needs to be directed at the main aetiological factors responsible for the wound. To determine which factors play an important role in a particular patient's case, it is essential to obtain a thorough and relevant medical history of the patient. A multitude of factors such as: age; past operations; possible post-operative complications; chronic medical conditions or comorbidities, such as signs or symptoms of arterial or venous insufficiency or other vascular disorders; anaemia; diabetes mellitus or other endocrine or metabolic disorders; nephropathy; neuropathy; hepatic dysfunction; connective tissue disorders; osteomyelitis; human immunodeficiency virus (HIV); immobility; dementia; malignancies; stress; current medication; psychosocial and socio-economic circumstances, on their own, or in combination, contribute to the non-healing nature and the longevity of wounds. A comprehensive medical history is essential to assist in determining which aetiologies may be excluded, and which should be explored further.

Careful attention should be given to the medical history, as it can provide important clues and indications that are useful and save time when making a diagnosis and in the subsequent treatment. Conversely, a badly taken, or brief medical history, may prove costly later on in terms of outcomes, and expenditure of time and resources.

Examination

When faced with a new patient with a wound, the initial focus should be on the patient as a whole. The first step is to obtain a general status followed by a more in-depth examination, directed at those areas relevant to the findings in the patient's medical history, and, only thereafter, move on to examining the wound and its surrounding skin. While most healthcare professionals dealing with wounds are skilled at examining a wound and its surrounding tissues, this is not necessarily the case when it comes to assessing the patient as a whole. For the reasons previously stated, it is important that the physician should be involved in the initial examination.

Investigations

Investigations, such as laboratory tests, radiographs, colour duplex scans or biopsies can be challenging and even painful to the patient. They are also costly in terms of both direct and indirect costs, such as time for both the patient and the institution involved. Consequently, every investigation undertaken should be necessary, and the questions for which the tests are intended to provide answers should be clearly formulated — for example, can a particular disease state be confirmed or excluded? It should be emphasised that interpretation of the results and the treatment choice must be based on the clinical findings, and not exclusively the radiograph or the laboratory tests which have a secondary role to these findings.

Diagnosis

Wound diagnosis is complex. There is no single factor which will lead to the diagnosis. Diagnosis is a synthesis of a careful medical history, clinical, laboratory and other findings and diagnostic tests, as well as possible indicators obtained from the earlier management of the wound and the outcomes achieved. Making an accurate diagnosis requires good patient and wound assessment skills, together with an understanding of how to interpret the results and findings of the examinations and investigations.

Indicators

The choice of indicators for success or failure of the treatment plan depends on the realistic expected outcome, and the time-frame in which this outcome is expected to be achieved. For example, in the healing of an acute wound in an otherwise healthy individual, it is likely that complete closure by re-epithelialisation of the wound, following a predictable pattern, is achievable in a reasonable time. In this case, re-epithelialisation and healing without complications is the indicator of an accurate diagnosis and an appropriate subsequent wound management plan. When the process is more lengthy and complex, or when it may not be realistic to expect healing as an outcome, it is important to define other indicators to evaluate the progress of the wound and treatment plan. Such indicators could, for instance, be reduction of wound size, decreased pain, increased intervals between dressing changes, reduced oedema, or management of odour. The indicator serves as a means of assessing the appropriateness of the treatment plan, and the accuracy of the working diagnosis. Thus, if the wound size is not decreasing in an uncomplicated venous leg ulcer treated with compression therapy, this may be an indicator of an incorrect working diagnosis, or that other complications have developed, such as infection, and it may be worth undertaking a complete reassessment and new examination of the patient.

Case histories illustrating the use of HEIDI

The following five case histories show the benefit of HEIDI as a framework for a structured approach in the management of a patient with a wound. This section also illustrates some of the reasons for non-healing wounds, or complications developing in patients attending our clinics.

Case history one

A fifty-three-year-old woman presented to her GP's surgery with a leg ulcer on her right leg below the medial malleolus. It had been present for more than six weeks. In the medical history she had a deep vein thrombosis (DVT), and a previous leg ulcer on the same leg, diagnosed as a venous leg ulcer. It had been successfully treated, and healed after a period of eleven weeks with compression therapy provided by the district nurse. The patient's notes indicated that this had taken place approximately one and a half years earlier. The notes also showed that the patient suffered from slightly raised cholesterol, kept under control with diet, was not obese, smoked about ten cigarettes per day, and her ankle brachial pressure index (ABPI) was normal.

Upon examination, the new ulcer measured 1.0cm x 1.6cm in size; it was shallow with a slightly sloughy wound base, well-defined borders, healthy looking surrounding skin, apart from some areas of atrophie blanche. The patient described the wound as painful.

The working diagnosis of a recurrent venous ulcer was made, and graduated sustained compression therapy was started. Four weeks later, the patient visited the local surgery complaining of severe ulcer pain. On inspection, the surrounding skin looked somewhat red; the ulcer had increased in size to 1.5cm x 2.2cm, the ulcer bed was covered with slough and there was a slight odour. Based on these findings the ulcer was diagnosed as infected and the patient was prescribed penicillin for fourteen days by her GP. Due to pain, the district nurse changed the compression from a four-layer bandage system to a modified compression system. Two weeks later, the situation had improved in that the patient was experiencing less pain, there seemed to be no odour, and the ulcer bed was less sloughy. However, the size remained unchanged. These findings suggested that the infection had been successfully treated and a four-layer bandage system was restarted as recommended in the local guidelines on treatment for venous leg ulcers. When the district nurse contacted the GP four weeks later, she felt limited progress was being made as the ulcer remained painful, seemed to be deteriorating, and the patient was non-compliant with the compression therapy. At this point, the patient was referred to our wound clinic.

The wound care specialist nurse and the physician in the clinic interviewed and examined the patient using HEIDI as a basis.

History

The medical history was mainly as reported before. However, when asked about her family history, the patient said that her father had died of a heart attack when he was in his seventies, her mother suffers from non-insulin dependent diabetes mellitus (NIDDM), high blood pressure and angina, and, while her older brother is healthy, her younger sister suffers from high blood pressure.

When further questioned about the pain she was experiencing, she described claudication-like pain and stated that lately she had been experiencing more pain at night time when resting in bed.

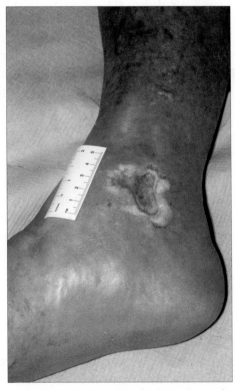

Figure 1.2: Example of a leg ulcer of mixed arterial and venous origin over medial malleolus of the right foot

Examination

The patient's overall general status seemed normal apart from a raised blood pressure of 160/100.

When examining her legs, palpable foot pulses were present bilaterally, the legs were somewhat pale, with some dusky red or blue areas on the right foot, and, on the same leg, patches of atrophie blanche, hyperpigmentation and lipodermatosclerosis were noted. The wound measured 1.8cm x 2.1cm and was shallow; the wound bed was pale with some areas of slough; there was little exudate, and the wound margins were well-defined.

Investigations

The ABPI was recorded as 0.7 in the right leg and 0.85 in the left leg.

Based on the above medical history and findings, the patient was sent for an arterial and a venous duplex scan of the right lower limb, in addition to the routine blood tests such as full blood count, liver function tests, urea + electrolytes, as well as glycosylated haemoglobin.

Diagnosis

Based on the medical history, initial examination and ABPI, the ulcer was diagnosed as a leg ulcer of mixed venous and arterial origin. Subsequently, the patient's compression regime was changed to a two-layer system of differing lengths of elasticated tubular bandage, and a simple non-adhesive dressing.

Indicators

Decrease in pain and wound size were established as the indicators for successful treatment while awaiting results from the investigations. A letter was written to the GP suggesting that the patient's blood pressure be monitored.

At the next visit, four weeks later, the results of the investigations were available. The blood tests were all normal. The venous duplex scan was normal indicating recanalisation, and adequate blood flow in the deep venous system; however, the arterial duplex scan showed a small occluded segment in the right superficial femoral artery.

There was less pain in the ulcer, and the night pain as well as claudication were unchanged. The ulcer status and status of the surrounding skin remained essentially unchanged. The patient also reported continuous raised blood pressure levels for which the GP was considering drug treatment.

After this visit, based on HEIDI, the wound treatment continued and the patient was referred to a vascular surgeon for assessment and possible revascularisation.

After a successful angioplasty (before which the patient had stopped smoking), the ulcer healed in approximately nine weeks.

Arterial disease

Arterial disease, such as arteriosclerosis, is a common finding in an elderly patient. The extent of the disease depends on factors such as genetic predisposition; presence of other chronic disease states, such as diabetes mellitus; and lifestyle, including diet and smoking. The narrowing or total occlusion of the arterial vessels as a consequence of the disease compromises the increased blood flow required for tissue repair and regeneration. Hence, patients suffering from the disease will, to a degree (dependent on the stage of the disease), be predisposed to poor healing and, in severe cases, to tissue necrosis and ulceration.

Diagnosis of arterial insufficiency in the absence of a previous diagnosis may be difficult, or even missed, as the reason for a non-healing wound. The patient history in this case is the most important factor in diagnosing arterial disease. Arteriosclerosis does not occur in isolation in one part of the body, and may well be present in one location before symptoms occur elsewhere. An indication of arteriosclerosis in the family history, or in the medical history in an area not directly related to the wound, or in the overall examination, should alert the clinician to make the appropriate examinations and investigations to determine whether arterial disease can be excluded as a reason for possible deteriorating or non-healing wounds.

Resting the limb after exercise relieves intermittent claudication or cramp-like pain caused by inadequate oxygen supply to the muscles. It is important to note that the location of the pain is dependent on the level of the occlusion, and, although this is most often experienced in the calf muscles, cramp-like pain higher up, for instance in the buttocks, should not be neglected. Rest pain is associated with severe ischaemia. Night pain may be present and is caused by position-induced poor blood supply and, typically, relieved by pending the limb in question.

Vascular intervention to improve perfusion to the affected area is required for healing and to avoid further complications and deterioration.

Case history two

A sixty-nine-year-old man had been treated in our leg ulcer clinic for eighteen months. The initial diagnosis of venous leg ulceration had been confirmed by colour flow duplex imaging. The ulcer was treated with sustained graduated compression. Complete wound healing had been established as an appropriate goal, and markers of healing as indicators for successful treatment. The wound initially showed progress to healing, but later became a static non-healing wound. Because the healed areas were breaking down repeatedly, the patient was seen by a physician who interviewed and re-examined the patient using HEIDI.

History

Overall, the patient had no significant medical history, apart from varicose veins and a venous ulcer four years earlier in the same leg, which had healed in ten weeks with compression therapy. He was a non-smoker, was not on any medication, and had no known allergies.

Examination

The overall medical status was normal apart from bilateral varicose veins. The ulcer was located over the anterior aspect of the left lower leg, and showed no obvious features of an unusual pathology. It was shallow, had well-defined borders, flat, sloping edges, islands of granulation tissue, and some evidence of re-epithelialisation.

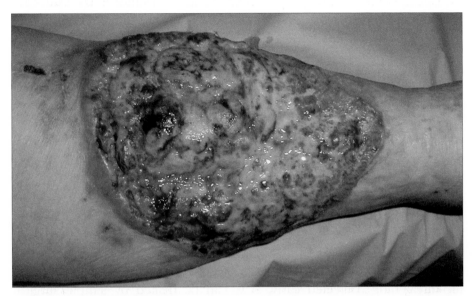

Figure 1.3: Example of a squamous cell carcinoma (Marjolin's ulcer) on the anterior aspect of the leg

Investigations

Based on the non-significant findings and observation of repeated breakdown of granulation tissue, a punch biopsy was performed.

Diagnosis

Based on the findings, medical history and observations, Marjolin's ulcer was established as a working diagnosis.

The histology revealed the ulcer to be a poorly differentiated, invasive squamous cell carcinoma (SCC). The patient was subsequently referred to a dermatological surgeon. He had an excision of the lesion with 1cm margins, and the defect was covered with a split-thickness graft. The margins were clear on histological examination. It is also important to note that he had no regional lymphadenopathy.

Indicators

Complete wound healing was established as the indicator for successful treatment. The patient subsequently healed and has remained so since.

Squamous cell carcinoma

Squamous cell carcinoma is one of the most common skin tumour types. An ulcer may be the first symptom of the tumour. It may also, however, develop as a complication of an ulcer of longer duration, as in the case of the patient described above. This type of ulcer was first described by the French surgeon, J Marjolin in 1828, hence its name.

A delay in diagnosis of SCC could lead to local destruction and deeper invasion, necessitating a more aggressive approach, and can result in loss of the affected limb. Furthermore, a SCC which has metastasised can be life-threatening. Detected early, SCC can be treated by simple surgical excision. The timely decision by the wound care specialist nurse in charge of the patient to bring in the physician to re-examine the patient, and to verify the accuracy of the initial diagnosis — in this case of a non-healing ulcer — led to the successful outcome and healing of this wound.

Case history three

A sixty-two-year-old man with NIDDM, neuropathy and an interdigital ulcer on his right foot, between the first and second toes, presented to the diabetic foot clinic for his follow-up appointment. He explained that he did not wear his special footwear because his right first toe was very swollen, and he had two days earlier been diagnosed with gout, for which he was now receiving medication. He also said that he had been visiting the diabetes specialist nurse as his glucose control had been poor during the previous week.

History

This was the patient's first ulcer which had been present for approximately eighteen weeks, during which time he had been cared for by the district nurse and the community podiatrist. The ulcer had remained static for the last four weeks. The patient had good glucose control, and good vascularity had been established in the limb in question. Furthermore, the patient's medical history was non-significant and had not revealed any reasons to suspect compromised healing.

Complete wound healing was the goal for treatment, and markers for healing as indicators for successful treatment. Initially, the wound had progressed to healing, but had remained static during the last month.

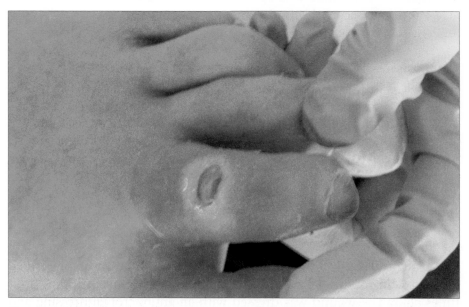

Figure 1.4: Example of a 'sausage toe', acute osteomyelitis in a patient with diabetes

Examination

The patient was somewhat obese but his normal blood pressure was normal. The left foot was ulcer free and the foot pulses were readily palpable in both feet. The feet looked well cared for in general. Upon examination of the right foot, the physician made note of a warm, red and swollen first toe. There was no sensation or pain. The swelling and configuration of the toe resembled a 'sausage toe', which, in a patient with diabetes, is indicative of osteomyelitis. After debridement, on probing, the wound did not probe to bone. There was, however, purulent discharge from the wound which bled easily on contact.

Investigations

The patient had blood tests to measure his inflammatory markers and a plain radiograph of his right foot to look for evidence of osteomyelitis.

The patient's surgery was contacted for the results of the blood tests that they had performed when gout had been diagnosed. The serum uric acid value had been 0.42mm/L.

Diagnosis

Based on the clinical findings supported by the patient's medical history, and the inconclusive laboratory value for uric acid, the working diagnosis was osteomyelitis.

Indicators

The patient was asked to stop the gout medication and was prescribed ciprofloxacin 500mg twice daily, combined with clindamycin 300mg, four times daily. The wound was dressed with an antimicrobial dressing and daily dressing changes were arranged with the district nurse. The patient was asked to rest his leg and stay off his feet as much as possible.

Decreasing temperature, swelling and redness were established as indicators of accurate diagnosis and an appropriate treatment plan.

Two days later, the blood test results showed raised inflammatory markers, notably a C-reactive protein (CRP) of 62; the radiograph showed some changes but, while osteomyelitis was not confirmed, it could not be excluded as the reason for the changes seen in the radiograph. Previous radiographs were not available for comparison.

When the patient was seen two weeks later, the 'sausage toe' appearance was no longer evident; however, there was still some purulent discharge from the wound. Six weeks after the initiation of the antibiotics, the purulent discharge had disappeared, the ulcer had somewhat decreased in size, and the inflammatory markers were normal.

The patient has since developed yet another setback: wound infection. The wound has, however, continued to decrease in size and, at the time of writing, has almost healed.

Infection in the diabetic foot

People with diabetes are more prone to infection. Infection in a diabetic foot is a serious complication of diabetic foot ulceration. If infection is present, it is to be treated as a matter of priority. It is potentially limb-threatening, and always requires urgent diagnostic and therapeutic attention. Microorganisms are present in all wounds, and the consensus is that infection should be diagnosed clinically, not based on swab cultures. The difficulty is that systemic manifestations, such as fever or leucocytosis, are often lacking and, therefore, the diagnosis is mostly based on local signs, such as purulent discharge, with local symptoms of inflammation (erythema, swelling, redness and warmth of the toe or foot). The presence of peripheral neuropathy means symptoms of pain are not always present. The nature of tissue involved, adequacy of arterial supply, and presence of systemic manifestations, determine the severity of the infection.

Aerobic gram-positive cocci (especially *Staphylococcus aureus*) are the predominant pathogens. Chronic, deep, and especially previously antibiotic-treated infections, are often polymicrobial, with gram-negative rods and anaerobic pathogens. Appropriately obtained cultures (tissue specimens obtained by biopsy, ulcer curettage, or aspiration), rather than swabs, may help to identify the causative organisms. Antibiotic therapy of infected foot wounds is usually initially empiric, and should always include coverage of gram-positive cocci. Broad-spectrum therapy is indicated for severe infections pending culture results, and antibiotic susceptibility data. Severity of infection, structures involved, adequacy of debridement, type of soft tissue cover, and wound vascularity, should all be considered when determining the duration of therapy. Subsequent therapy can be revised, if needed, based on the patient's clinical response and the culture results.

Most infections require some surgical treatment. This may range from debridement to incision and drainage, or, more extensive excision of necrotic tissues may be required. Early and careful follow-up of the effect of treatment is always required.

Osteomyelitis

About 50%–60% of serious foot infections are complicated by osteomyelitis. This can be difficult to diagnose. Plain radiography may be adequate in many cases, but magnetic resonance imaging (MRI) is more sensitive and specific. The ability to probe to bone in the base of an ulcer has been shown in patients with diabetes to have a predictive value of 89% for osteomyelitis. The appearance of a 'sausage toe' has also been shown as a sign indicating the presence of osteomyelitis in the diabetic foot. Treatment for osteomyelitis depends on the severity, but may include a long-term (six weeks or more) course of antibiotics, either oral or intravenous, and may require hospitalisation. There is also evidence that surgery to debride the infected bone can be successful in treating osteomyelitis. Amputation, ultimately, may be required in severe cases.

Gout

Gout is characterised by raised levels of uric acid in the blood, followed by the deposition of urate crystals in joints or soft tissue. It typically presents as a mono-arthritis with an acute onset. The first metatarso-phalangeal joint is the most affected joint, and the onset is typically characterised by local irritation and aching, followed by swelling; the affected area becomes red, hot, shiny, and extremely painful. The pain is often described as 'the worst ever experienced'. After twenty-four hours inflammation is maximal, resolving slowly over the next few weeks, often with itching and flaking of the skin overlying the affected area.

Uric acid is the end product of purine metabolism, and humans and higher apes lack urease, an enzyme which degrades uric acid. Two-thirds of the uric acid formed each day is eliminated in the gastrointestinal tract or kidneys. In most people with gout (75%–90%), clearance of uric acid by the kidney is significantly reduced. Primary gout develops most often in men between thirty and sixty years of age.

The major causes for gout are:

- idiopathic (often familial)
- obesity
- alcohol
- renal disease
- drugs, eg. thiazides (diuretics), aspirin
- hypothyroidism
- lymphoproliferative and myeloproliferative disorders
- severe psoriasis
- hypertension
- polycythaemia
- a diet high in purine content.

Secondary gout usually results from chronic diuretic therapy and presents in older subjects, often older than sixty-five years.

In people aged sixty-five to seventy-four years in the UK, the prevalence of gout is approximately 50/1000 in men, and 9/1000 in women.

Case history four

A sixty-seven-year-old lady was referred to our wound clinic by her GP with a four-month history of a painful ulcer on her right medial malleolus.

History

The patient was fit and had no history of any relevant clinical disorder, including DVT or cardiac problems. She was a non-smoker and there were no known drug allergies in her medical history. During the initial examination, it was noted that she had some lymphoedema, and while the dorsalis pedis pulse was palpable, the posterior tibial pulse was not. The ulcer was superficial and surrounded by eczema. Her ABPI was normal and she was treated with a mild steroid ointment for the eczema, and graduated compression with a simple dressing covering the ulcer. Four months later, the ulcer healed. However, three months after healing, the ulcer recurred in the same location.

On presentation to the wound clinic no changes were noted, neither in her medical history nor in her medical status, and the same treatment as before was initiated. The ulcer remained static for six months, at which point she developed an infection and the ulcer increased in size.

At the next visit, the ulcer remained painful and static and there were no indications of healing or improvement. The patient was re-assessed. Further review of the medical history revealed nothing new, and the clinical status was equally unchanged, apart from the notes on the level of pain from the ulcer site. This was noted as mild and tolerable during the initial ulceration, and an increase in pain level seemed to be the only change which had occurred during the past year of follow-up. The question of a possible vasculitic origin of the ulcer was therefore raised, and an ulcer biopsy and blood tests were taken to detect autoimmune antibodies; inflammatory markers were also undertaken.

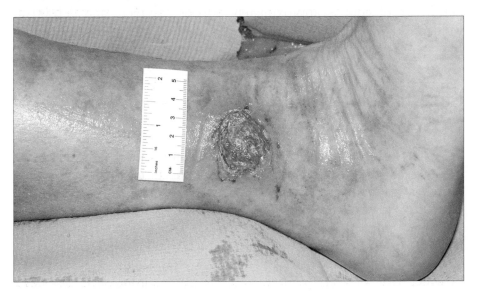

Figure 1.5: Example of a vasculitic ulcer in a patient with rheumatoid arthritis

Two weeks later when all the results were available, the patient was again seen in the wound clinic. The biopsy result was normal, the full blood count (FBC) was normal, however, anti–ENA, anti-Ro, and anti-La were detected, together with a strongly positive RA test and anti-nuclear antibodies. As these results are strongly indicative of an autoimmune disorder, the patient was referred to a rheumatologist for further investigations and treatment of the underlying disorder. The follow-up of the patient's leg ulcer continues in the wound clinic, while awaiting advice on the correct diagnosis and treatment of the autoimmune disorder from the rheumatologist.

Vasculitis

Vasculitis is a general term for a group of diseases that involve inflammation in blood vessels, with resulting damage and narrowing or occlusion of the vessel in question. This, inevitably, leads to poor blood supply and may lead to ischaemic necrosis of the affected area. Blood vessels of all sizes may be affected, from the large vessels to the capillaries. The size of blood vessel affected varies according to the specific type of vasculitis. On the skin vasculitis may manifest as ulcers which, consequently, are called vasculitic ulcers. This type of ulceration is usually painful, with a punched-out appearance, presenting with a necrotic wound bed, often with purple-red edges. There may be black necrotic areas and blisters, and the surrounding skin is often oedematous with purpuric spots, or purple macules; sometimes pigmentation is present.

Vasculitic ulcers are typically seen in patients with autoimmune disorders. Autoimmune disorders are caused by the body producing an immune response against its own tissues. The cause is not known, but is often the result of multiple circumstances: for example, a genetic predisposition triggered by an infection. Sex hormones may play a role and there is a higher prevalence of autoimmune disorders in women than in men. It has been estimated that nearly 79% of autoimmune disease patients are women.

Autoimmune disorders affect many organs or tissues and are called systemic autoimmune disorders; or they affect a single organ or tissue, in which case they are referred to as localised autoimmune disorders. The following table contains a list of the most common autoimmune disorders with the affected organ(s) or tissue(s) in parenthesis.

Table 1.1: The most common autoimmune disorders	
Systemic autoimmune disorders	Localised autoimmune disorders
Rheumatoid arthritis (joints, less commonly lung, skin)	Type I diabetes mellitus (pancreas islets)
Systemic lupus erythematosus (SLE) (skin, joints, kidneys, heart, brain, red blood cells, other)	Hashimoto's thyroiditis, Grave's disease (thyroid)
Scleroderma (skin, intestine, less commonly lung)	Celiac disease, Chrohn's disease, ulcerative colitis (GI tract)
Sjögren's syndrome (salivary glands, tear glands, joints)	Guillan-Barré syndrome (CNS)
Goodpasture's syndrome (lungs, kidneys)	Addison's disease (adrenal gland)
Wegener's granulomatosis (sinuses, lungs, kidneys)	Primary biliary sclerosis, sclerosing cholangitis, autoimmune hepatitis (liver)
Polymyalgia rheumatica (large muscle groups)	Raynaud's phenomenon (fingers, toes, nose, ears)
Temporal arteritis/giant cell arteritis (arteries of the head and neck)	

In some cases, the antibodies are not directed at a specific organ. This is the case in antiphospholipid syndrome, where the antibodies may react with clotting proteins in the blood, and lead to thrombosis of the vessel concerned.

Vasculitis is diagnosed by a combination of findings in the medical history, results of patient and wound examination, together with results from blood tests for antibodies indicating autoimmune disease, and the histopathological results of a wound biopsy.

Case history five

A seventy-one-year-old, retired midwife, presented to our wound clinic having been referred by her GP because of the deteriorating condition of her leg ulcers.

History

The patient's main complaint was weeping infected ulcers on her left leg. The condition had started about eighteen months earlier with a small ulcer in the area of the medial malleolus. This had been diagnosed as a recurrent venous ulcer, and the patient had been treated with modified compression and an adhesive foam dressing. The district nurse called on the patient twice a week. Over the previous three months the ulcer had begun to deteriorate and the surrounding skin was breaking down. A new area of ulceration had appeared in the gaiter area, originally over the shin, but later developed into an almost circumferential ulcer. The patient found her condition painful and irritating. She was particularly bothered by the burning, painful itching, the odour, and the exudate which had increased despite an increase in her usual dose of diuretics. The patient suffered from cardiac insufficiency, high blood pressure, and diet-controlled diabetes mellitus. She was a non-smoker and suffered from no known allergies. Her current medication was bendrofluazide 5mg daily, digoxin 125mcg daily, and paracetamol as required.

Examination

The patient was somewhat obese; her pulse, blood pressure and heart sounds were normal. The abnormal findings related to her legs. Both ankles and feet were swollen; the skin on the left leg was wet, with extensive areas of broken skin and eczema. There was a strong odour present and the bright green colour of the sloughy areas, as well as the debris on the dressings suggested a pseudomonal infection. Around the areas of the upper border of the compression bandages there were scratch marks, and the patient admitted to having scratched these areas because of the severe irritation. Due to the oedema, the pedal pulses were not palpable. On the right leg, just above the medial malleolus, there was a shallow, somewhat sloughy ulcer, measuring 1.5cm x 2.2cm.

Investigations

An ABPI was attempted but, due to the swelling and pain, this was not successfully completed. No further investigations were carried out.

Diagnosis

The working diagnosis was established as hydrostatic eczema complicated by a local bilateral pseudomonas infection.

Indicators

The patient was prescribed potassium permanganate soaks for ten days, followed by ten days of treatment on alternate days to treat the pseudomonal infection and to decrease the levels of exudate. A potent steroid ointment was also prescribed, which was to be applied daily to the eczematous areas for two weeks, followed by a moderately potent steriod ointment daily for a further two weeks. The ulcer was covered with a simple non-adhesive dressing, and two layers of tubular bandage were applied to provide compression.

There was a decrease in the amount of exudate, irritation and eczema, as well as a decrease in odour, indicating correct diagnosis and successful treatment.

The patient was cared for in the community and seen in the wound clinic three weeks later. During this visit no odour was present, the eczema had dramatically decreased, and there was neither irritation nor pain present. The ulcer on the right leg measured 1.0cm x 1.3cm. The ABPIs were measured bilaterally and were found to be normal. The patient was prescribed graduated sustained compression bilaterally. A change of dressings was recommended three times a week, and the moderately potent steroid ointment was to continue to be applied at each dressing change for another two weeks, after which it was to be changed to a mild steroid ointment. Another visit was arranged six weeks later and, at this visit, the skin was intact bilaterally, and the leg ulcer had healed. The patient was measured up for class II compression stockings, and was to continue to use a moderately potent steroid ointment. A moisturiser was recommended for use on any dry or inflamed patches.

Gravitational eczema

Swollen ankles are a common complaint and may be the result of local, regional or systemic disease. In general, chronic swelling of one leg is more likely to be local, whereas bilateral swelling usually has a systemic cause, such as cardiac failure, but can be due to a local or lymphatic problem.

Gravitational eczema is an eruption that develops as a consequence of venous hypertension. It characteristically originates around the 'gaiter' region of the lower leg. Venous ulceration is not essential for its development and the mechanism for its cause is still unknown. It often complicates the management of leg ulcers of venous or mixed origin, but not other types of leg ulcers. The prevalence of gravitational eczema among patients with venous leg ulcers has been reported to be as high as 47% in a hospital-based study, and 65% in a large community-based study. Approximately 40% of venous leg ulcer patients attending our clinics develop gravitational eczema. It may affect any age and affects both sexes equally.

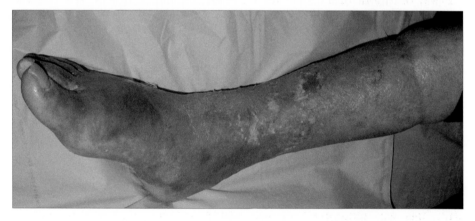

Figure 1.6: Example of gravitational eczema on the right leg

Gravitational eczema is a clinical diagnosis. Patients usually experience itching, but may describe sensations such as burning or stinging. Examination should reveal excoriation, erythema with unclear (diffuse) edge, scaling, dryness or weeping to varying degrees, depending on its severity. In severe gravitational eczema, the skin may be eroded and give the appearance of having multiple small ulcers.

It is often associated with considerable discomfort for the patient. In acute gravitational eczema, superficial oedema and weeping may lead to maceration and erosion of the skin. Its presence increases the risk of infection and of developing allergic contact dermatitis. It is widely believed that the use of potent topical corticosteroids to treat gravitational eczema impair leg ulcer healing.

Differentiating gravitational eczema from cellulitis may be difficult. In contrast to gravitational eczema, cellulitis is associated with bright, confluent, well-demarcated erythema, which is characteristically warm and extremely tender. It should also be noted that cellulitis and gravitational eczema could occur together. The following table which provides some of the characteristics of the two conditions is intended to assist in the differential diagnosis.

Table 1.2: Characteristics of gravitational eczema and cellulitis	
Gravitational eczema	Cellulitis
Patient afebrile	Patient unwell/febrile
Pruritus or burning sensation	Soreness, burning, tenderness
Diffuse erythema	Erythema demarcated
No lymphadenopathy	Lymphadenopathy
Excoriations of skin	Portal of entry
Normal whole blood count (WBC)	Elevated whole blood count (WBC)

Conclusion

According to a consensus statement issued by the International Committee on Wound Management:

> *Wound management is the pursuit of the permanent, functional and aesthetic healing of the patient's wound through the promotion of physiological healing and the prevention or elimination of factors — whether local, systemic or external — that disturb healing.*

Ideally, the management of patients with wounds requires referral to a multidisciplinary team with knowledge in wound care. The size, composition, and the profession in charge of this team may vary. The prerequisite to successful treatment outcomes is a correct diagnosis, based on an in-depth understanding of the underlying pathologies responsible for the disease in question. Patients with wounds may often suffer from several underlying health problems, all, or many of which, could affect the origin of the wound, as well as the healing process. This can make the assessment and diagnosis complex. Therefore, a physician, as a member of the multidisciplinary team caring for patients with wounds, has a leading role to play in making the initial diagnosis and holistic assessment, as well as any subsequent modifications to the working diagnosis. A structured approach, such as HEIDI, has been shown to be successful and is routinely used in, and recommended by, our wound clinic.

Bibliography

Bodenheimer T, MacGregor K, Stothart N (2005) Nurses as leaders in chronic care. *Br Med J* **330**: 612–13

Boulton AJM, Connor H, Cavanagh PR (2000) *The Foot in Diabetes*. Wiley, Chichester

Callum MJ (1989) *Chronic Leg Ulceration: The Lothian and Forth Valley Study.* ChM Thesis. University of Dundee

Enoch S, Miller DR, Price PE, Harding KG (2004) Early diagnosis is vital in the management of squamous cell carcinomas associated with chronic non-healing ulcers: a case series and review of the literature. *Int Wound J* **1**(3)

Enoch S, Price P (2004) Should alternative endpoints be considered to evaluate outcomes in chronic recalcitrant wounds? Available online at: http//:www.worldwidewounds.com

Falanga V, Phillips T, Harding KG, Moy R, Peerson L (2000) *Text Atlas of Wound Management*. Martin Dunitz, London: 310

Glasziou P, Irwig L, Mant D (2005) Monitoring in chronic disease: a rational approach. *Br Med J* **330**: 644–6

Gorman PW, Davis KR, Donnelly R (2000) Swollen lower limb — 1: General assessment and deep vein thrombosis. In: Donnelly R, London NJ, eds. *ABC of Arterial and Venous Disease*. BMJ Books, London: 46–9

Groves T, Wagner E (2005) High quality care for people with chronic diseases. *Br Med J* **330**: 609–10

Harding KG (2000) Non-healing wounds:r ecalcitrant, chronic, or not understood? *Ostomy Wound Management* **46**(1-A suppl)

Harding KG, Morris HL, Patel GK(2002) Science, medicine and the future: healing chronic wounds. *Br Med J* **324**: 160–3

Hess CT, Trent JT (2004) Incorporating laboratory values in chronic wound management. *Adv Skin Wound Care* **17**: 378–86

International Working Group on the Diabetic Foot (1999) *International Consensus on the Diabetic Foot*. International Working Group on the Diabetic Foot. ISBN 90-9012716-x

Jeffcoate WJ, Harding KG (2003) Diabetic foot ulcers. *Lancet* **361**: 1545–51

Jeffcoate WJ, Price P, Harding KG (2004) Wound healing and treatments for people with diabetic foot ulcers. *Diabetes/Metabolism Res Rev* **20**(suppl 1): S78–S89

Lab Test available online a: http://www.labtestsonline.org

Lazarus GS, Cooper DM, Knighton DR *et al* (1994) Definitions and guidelines for assessment of wounds and evaluation of healing. *Arch Dermatol* **130**: 489–93

Lipsky BA, van Baal JG, Harding KG, guest editors (2004) Diabetic foot infection: epidemiology, pathophysiology, diagnosis, treatment and prevention. *Clin Infect Dis* **39**(Suppl 2): S75–S139

London NJ, Nash R (2000) Varicose veins. In: Donnelly R, London NJ, eds. *ABC of Arterial and Venous Disease*. BMJ Books, London: 42–5

London NJ, Donelly R (2000) Ulcerated lower limb. In: Donnelly R, London NJ, eds. *ABC of Arterial and Venous Disease*. BMJ Books, London: 53–5

Mekkes JR, Loots MAM, Van Der Wal AC, Bos JD (2003) Cause, investigation and treatment of leg ulceration. *Br J Dermatol* **148**: 388–401

National Institute for Clinical Excellence (2004) *National Collaborating Centre for Primary Care. Type 2 Diabetes Prevention and Management of Foot Problems*. NICE, London

Paramsothy Y, Collins M, Smith AG (1988) Contact dermatitis in patients with leg ulcers. *Contact Dermatitis* **18**: 30–6

Patel GK, Llewellyn M et al (2001) Gravitational eczema: not all bad news. *Br J Dermatol* **147**(62): 25–7

Patel GK, Llewellyn M, Harding KG (2001) Managing gravitational eczema and contact dermatitis. *Br J Community Nurs* **6**: 394–406

Quartey-Papafio CM (1999) Importance of distinguishing between cellulitis and varicose eczema of the leg. *Br Med J* **318**: 1672–3

Sanders LJ (1994) Diabetes mellitus:prevention of amputation. *J Am Podiatr Med Assoc* **84**: 322–8

Savage C, Harper L, Cockwell P, Adu D, Howie AJ (2000) Vasculitis. In: Donnelly R, London NJ, eds. *ABC of Arterial and Venous Disease*. BMJ Books, London: 38–41

Stadelmann WK, Digenis AG, Tobin GR (1998) Impediments to wound healing. *Am J Surg* **176**: 39S–47S

The Wound Programme (1992) Centre for Medical Education, Dundee and Perspective, London. ISBN 1871 749 239

Wagner EH, Austin BT, Hindmarsh M, Schaefer J, Bonomi A (2001) Improving chronic illness care:translating evidence into action. *Health Affairs* **20**: 64–78

Wortmann RL (1994) Gout and other disorders of purine metabolism. In: Isselbacher, Braunwald, Wilson *et al*, eds. *Harrison's Principles of Internal Medicine*, 13th edn. McGraw-Hill Inc: 2079–88

CHAPTER 2

A REVIEW OF DIFFERENT WOUND TYPES AND THEIR PRINCIPLES OF MANAGEMENT

Pam Cooper

Introduction

Wounds can be categorised into many different groups and sub-groups according to their wide and varied pathologies. However, it is possible to categorise most wounds healing by secondary intention into the following six categories; pressure ulcers, leg ulcers, diabetic foot ulcers, trauma wounds, surgical wounds and complex wounds. Before embarking on any plan of care, it is vital that the practitioner understands the cause of the wound and considers into which of the above categories the wound fits. An understanding of the basic principles of each type of wound is also essential to ensure well-informed clinical decision-making.

The three Wound Continuums, Healing, Infection and Exudate (*Chapter 3, p. 60*) provide a framework for assessing a wound in a systematic manner. However, it is essential that when assessing a wound, the practitioner understands the underlying pathology of the wound to accurately inform clinical decision-making. Such an understanding, combined with key management principles for the wound, be it a pressure, leg, or diabetic foot ulcer, can greatly enhance the level of care provided. For example, in the case of a pressure ulcer, removing the cause, eg. an inappropriate seat cushion, can prevent further damage and facilitate healing.

This chapter presents a brief overview of common wound types, and the key principles for their management.

Pressure ulcers

Pressure ulcers (pressure sores, decubitus ulcers, bedsores) are areas of tissue death, usually located over a bony prominence, which have been caused by external forces of pressure, shear and friction (Allman, 1997). These may be further exacerbated by complications arising from the individual's physical condition, such as altered nutrition, excess moisture, etc (Maklebust, 1987).

* ❖ **Pressure** is the major causative factor in the development of pressure ulcers. The damage occurs when the body's soft tissue is compressed between a bony prominence and a hard surface, which occludes the blood supply, leading to tissue ischaemia and death.

* ❖ **Shear** usually occurs when the individual slides down the bed, the skeleton and close tissue move but the skin on the buttocks remains in the same place. This usually leads to the development of more extensive tissue damage.

* ❖ **Friction** occurs when two surfaces move or rub across one another, leading to superficial skin loss.

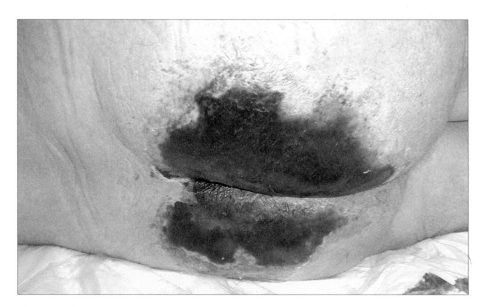

Figure 2.1: Pressure ulcer to sacrum

The care of those individuals who are either at risk of pressure ulcer development, or with existing pressure ulcers, should be based on prevention of pressure ulcers or the management/treatment of existing pressure ulcer damage. This approach should be holistic, focusing on the individual as a whole.

Physical assessment

* **General health:** Bliss (1990) suggests that acutely ill individuals are particularly vulnerable to the development of pressure ulcers, although the reasons for this are uncertain. If there has been a change in the individual's condition through illness, this should be considered when assessment of risk is carried out.

* **Age:** the majority of pressure ulcers recorded are found in the elderly, those over sixty-five years of age. This may be due to changes in their physical condition and skin. The skin loses its natural elasticity and becomes thinner, making it more susceptible to damage.

* **Reduced mobility:** this reduces the individual's ability to alter position and to relieve pressure, be it in bed or while sitting up, thus making them more susceptible to the effects of sustained pressure.

* **Nutritional status:** this impairs the elasticity of the skin, reducing its ability to sustain the effects of pressure, shear and friction without leading to tissue breakdown.

* **Incontinence:** it is now generally recognised that incontinence has a significant impact on the development of pressure ulcers, due to the combined effects of moisture, friction and pressure. Jordan *et al* (1977) found that 15.5% of patients with pressure ulcers were incontinent of urine, and 39.7% were incontinent of faeces.
    Skin has a mean pH of 5.5 which is slightly acidic. Both urine and faeces are alkaline in nature, therefore, if the individual is incontinent, there is an immediate chemical reaction. Ammonia is produced when microorganisms rupture urea from the urine. Although urinary ammonia alone is not a primary irritant, urine and faeces together increase the pH at the peri-anal area, prompting

the faecal irritant effect (Leyden _et al_, 1977; Berg, 1986). This is responsible for the dermatitis excoriation seen in individuals with incontinence (Fiers, 1996). The increase in moisture from episodes of incontinence, combined with bacterial and enzymatic activity, can cause the breakdown of vulnerable skin, due to an increased friction co-efficient, particularly in the very young or elderly.

❖ **Poor blood supply:** patients with evidence of poor blood supply, particularly to the peripheries such as the foot, have an increased risk of pressure damage. The effect of sustained low pressure on an already compromised limb can lead to the development of extensive tissue damage over a very short period of time. Particular attention should be paid when caring for these patients.

Risk assessment

To consider preventing pressure ulcers we must first determine an individual's risk of pressure ulcer development. All risk assessment tools are based on factors known to predispose an individual to pressure ulcer development, such as sustained pressure, reduced mobility, incontinence, poor nutrition, age, mental alertness and poor physical condition. There are a number of risk assessment tools available to select from; Norton (1962), Gosnell (1973), Towey and Erland (1988), Waterlow (1984) and Braden (1985). All of which have a research-based rationale dependent on their patient population. However, it should be remembered that they are to be used as an 'aide memoir' alongside clinical judgement and experience. Any intervention adopted following risk assessment should be clearly recorded in the individual's health records.

Skin inspection

It is essential that skin inspections are carried out to determine what is normal reactive hyperaemia, and what is abnormal non-blanching hyperaemia.

❖ **Reactive hyperaemia** – the characteristic bright flush of the skin associated with the release of pressure, a direct response to incoming blood.

❖ **Non-blanching hyperaemia** – there is no skin colour change when light finger pressure is applied, indicating an alteration to the blood supply and an initial sign of pressure damage.

Table 2.1 shows how to assess if the changes to the skin are a result of pressure damage.

Table 2.1: Skin assessment
Further examination of erythema should include the following:
● Apply light finger pressure to the area for ten seconds
● Release the pressure. If the area is white and then returns to its original colour, the area probably has an adequate blood supply. Observation should continue and preventative strategies should be employed
● If, on release of pressure, the area remains the same colour as before pressure was applied, it is an indication of the beginning of pressure ulcer development and preventative strategies should be employed
● If there is an alteration in skin colour (red, purple or black), or increased heat or swelling, it may imply underlying tissue breakdown. Frequency of assessment should be increased
● With dark skin pigmentation, pressure ulcer development will be indicated by areas where there is localised heat, or where there is damage, coolness, purple/black discoloration, localised oedema and induration

Pressure ulcer grading

If following skin inspection, pressure damage is observed, this should be recorded using an appropriate grading system. The grading of the pressure ulcer determines the degree of tissue damage, assisting the clinician to determine the type and level of clinical intervention required. Although this is not without a thorough wound assessment as well. There are a number of grading tools available which assess the degree of tissue involvement, namely:

- European Pressure Ulcer Advisory Panel (EPUAP, 2002) – A guide to pressure ulcer grading
- Stirling pressure sore severity scale (SPSSS, 1994)
- Torrance pressure sore grading scale (1983)
- Pressure ulcer scale for healing (PUSH, 2001).

Once the pressure ulcer has been graded, the individual or their carer is able to start the appropriate treatment and set up the correct interventions.

Table 2.2: Principles of management of pressure ulcers
• Prevention is better than treatment. If the individual is at risk of pressure ulcer development, ensure that appropriate preventative strategies have been adopted
• If a pressure ulcer has occurred, identify, remove, or treat the cause
• Treat the wound following the principles of the Wound Healing Continuum, based on accurate classification and wound assessment
• Ensure that the individual is cared for on an appropriate support surface while in bed and sitting up, according to the location of the pressure ulcer
• Ensure that the individual's underlying physical condition does not affect his/her ability to heal, ie. poor nutritional status

Positioning

Individuals at risk of, or with existing pressure ulcers, should have their position changed to reduce the effects of pressure. This should not be based on ritualistic practice, but on skin assessment and the individual's needs (Roycroft–Malone, 2000).

The use of turning regimes, such as the 30° tilt, has been effective at reducing tissue damage (Young, 2004) without the need to physically turn the individual. This is achieved not by moving or lifting the individual, but by using pillows to alter their position.

Individuals at risk of, or with pressure ulcers, should always be nursed on the appropriate support surfaces. Also, they should not be up for long periods, with evidence suggesting a maximum of one hour before returning to bed for a minimum of two hours (Defloor, 1999; Gebhardt and Bliss, 1994).

Equipment — mattresses and seating

Mattresses

Over recent years, the market has been filled with a wide variety of support surfaces designed to reduce the effects of pressure, shear and friction. These can be divided into two categories: static mattress systems and alternating/dynamic systems.

* **Static systems:** these are high quality cut foams, visco-elastic foams, or static air-filled systems. They reduce the effects of pressure by contouring to the individual's shape, redistributing the pressure across a much larger surface area. They do not require a power unit for operation.

* **Alternating/dynamic systems:** these provide alternating or low air-loss, which reduces the pressure at the individual's bony prominences. The alternating systems work by alternating their cells over a specific period of time. The vast majority of these beds will self-adjust to the individual's weight, although they have a minimum and maximum weight within which they operate. They are power activated.

Seating

* **Chairs:** individuals are at a greater risk of developing a pressure ulcer while sitting up, as 75% of their body weight is being transferred through the relatively small surface area of the buttocks (Günnewicht and Dunford, 2004). An individual at risk of pressure damage, who needs to be seated, should have an appropriate

cushion on their chair or wheelchair to offer protection to the pressure areas. If sitting in a chair, the height should be considered, as if the chair is either too low or too high, an increased pressure is placed on both the sacrum and the heels.

* **Cushions**: the range of cushions has increased, leading to the development of cut foams, visco-elastic foams, gel inserts, static and alternating air systems. The individual should be fitted for the appropriate cushion, considering height, weight and postural alignment. Occupational therapists, if available, may be able to help.

The management of pressure ulcers is often complex and fraught, with attention being focused on treating the wound. However, when caring for an individual with a pressure ulcer, the key prevention and management principles should be considered.

Leg ulcers

Chronic leg ulcers are a major health problem within the UK, primarily affecting the elderly patient population. It has been suggested that 80% of these are being cared for within the community environment (Cornwall _et al_, 1986), increasing the demands on already stretched resources.

A chronic leg ulcer is defined as an open lesion between the knee and the ankle joint that remains unhealed for at least four weeks (Scottish Intercollegiate Guidelines Network [SIGN], 1998).

The assessment of the individual and the leg ulcer should be comprehensive. The individual's co-morbidity must be assessed as this may greatly influence the treatment's aims and objectives. The assessment should consider if the leg ulcer is arterial, venous, or mixed in aetiology, and should also exclude factors such as rheumatoid arthritis and systemic vasculitis, as well as diabetic lesions.

Leg ulcer assessment

Historically, the most common method of leg ulcer assessment has been the traditional Doppler assessment. However, the technique requires considerable skill and expertise, which can prove difficult for nurses to maintain as the test is rarely requested. This has led to the work being carried out using pulse oximetry and the development of the Lanarkshire oximetry index (LOI).

Doppler assessment

Measurement of ankle brachial pressure ratio (index) (ABPI) by hand-held Doppler is essential in the assessment of chronic leg ulcers (SIGN, 1998). This is based on the Doppler probe being held over the vein, the blood pressure cuff being inflated, and once the Doppler signal disappears this is your recorded value. The brachial systolic pressure recorded in the arm is used as the baseline recording, and then the posterior tibial and dorsalis pedis are recorded in the feet.

The ABPI is calculated for each leg by dividing the highest ankle systolic pressure of each leg by the higher of the two brachial pressures (Jones, 2000).

$$\text{ABPI} = \frac{\text{ankle systolic pressure}}{\text{brachial systolic pressure}}$$

* Pressures of 0.5–0.8 indicate evidence of significant arterial impairment (0.5 = 50% reduction in arterial blood flow).
* Pressures of 0.6–0.7 may have reduced compression if it has been assessed and applied by an experienced trained leg ulcer care expert (Royal College of Nursing [RCN], 1998).
* Pressures of 0.8 and above are suitable for compression (RCN, 1998). Caution should be taken with patients with diabetes and in patients with arteriosclerosis, as abnormally high readings might be caused by calcified arteries (Pudner, 1998).

Lanarkshire oximetry index (LOI)

The Lanarkshire oximetry index uses the method of pulse oximetry to measure the oxygen saturation of haemoglobin in blood or tissue, by detecting the amount of infrared light absorbed. However, like Doppler, it also depends on the presence of pulsatile blood flow in the arteries. This is carried out in a similar method to Doppler with the use of a blood pressure cuff, but instead of trying to find vessels, the probe is placed on one of the investigating limb's digits. The cuff is inflated initially to 60mmHG, then inflated in 10mmHG increments with ten seconds between each increment. When the pulse is lost, the pressure reading one below is recorded. A baseline recording is carried out on the arm and then the legs are investigated. The LOI is calculated as: LOI = toe pressure divided by finger pressure. Studies have suggested that LOI is at least as effective as Doppler (Bianchi, 2005), but it may have limitations in individuals with grossly dystrophic toe nails, extreme cyanosis, or in conditions where peripheral vascular constriction is evident.

Below are four of the most prevalent types of lower extremity wounds encountered in clinical practice.

Venous leg ulcers

Chronic venous insufficiency is due to impaired drainage in the venous system, with subsequent venous hypertension. Common sites for venous leg ulcers are above the medial malleoli and above the lateral malleoli.

Visual assessment of the skin and lower leg

On inspection, venous leg ulcers tend to be shallow in appearance without punched out wound margins located above the malleoli. Classic signs of venous leg ulceration are:

❖ **Varicose veins:** these are a clear indication of chronic venous hypertension in the lower limb, which is usually due to damage of the vessels there. About 3% of individuals with varicose veins go on to develop venous leg ulcers (Morison and Moffat, 1994).

❖ **Ankle flare:** chronic venous hypertension can cause distension of the tiny veins in the medial aspect of the foot. On inspection, it presents as purple blood vessel distoration, often referred to as ankle flare.

❖ **Lipodermatosclerosis:** the characteristic brown staining of the lower leg is suggestive of chronic venous disease. This occurs later on as progressive deposits of fibrous tissue in the deep dermis and fat result in the woody induration of the gaiter area of the shin.

❖ **Atrophie blanche:** this is often associated with irregular pigmentation, and presents as white areas of extremely thin skin dotted with tiny tortuous blood vessels.

❖ **Eczema:** this is commonly known as stasis dermatitis, and may appear in the gaiter area.

Visual inspection of the limb and a diagnostic assessment, ie. Doppler or LOI, should confirm if the limb is venous in nature. Once correct diagnosis is determined, treatment can be established.

Treatment

Patients with venous ulceration (ABPI >0.8) should have some form of elastic graduated compression applied with a simple non-adherent dressing to the wound. This may be a multi-layered bandage system (SIGN, 1998) or some form of compression hosiery (Best Practice Statement for Compression Hosiery, 2005). Therapeutic compression should provide a minimum of 30mmHg–40mmHg pressure at the ankle.

Arterial leg ulcers

Arterial ulcers are less common than those caused by venous disease, but arterial insufficiency, if present, complicates the healing of the wound. Arterial ulcers are caused by an insufficient arterial blood supply to the lower limb, resulting in tissue ischaemia and necrosis. Atherosclerosis is by far the commonest cause of venous insufficiency. Atherosclerosis reduces the blood flow to the lower limbs, and the degree of ischaemia and symptoms experienced depend not only on the site of occlusion, but also on the circulation above and below the occlusion site. At rest, an individual may be able to tolerate occlusion without experiencing any significant symptoms. However, during exercise, the increased demand for oxygen which cannot be met, can lead to intermittent claudication so that the person has to stop and rest because of the lack of blood supply to the muscles.

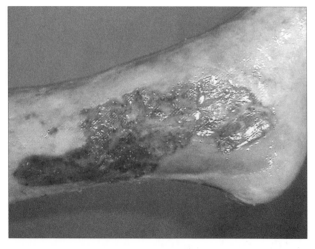

The majority of patients with claudication have an ABPI between 0.8 and 0.4,

Figure 2.2: Arterial leg ulcer

while patients with rest pain have an ABPI of <0.4 (Sumner, 1989).

Identified risk factors for arterial disease include smoking or tobacco use, hyperlipidaemia, diabetes, hypertension, obesity, advanced age, trauma, sickle cell disease, and cardiovascular disease.

Visual assessment of the skin and lower leg

When visually inspecting a limb thought to have an arterial ulcer, the following should be considered:

❖ **The ulcer itself:** arterial ulcers are mainly found on the anterior shin, over toe joints, over malleoli and under the heel. They usually present as a large area of tissue loss, often circumferential with deep wound edges, and are often described as a 'dog taking a bite'. They are usually very painful and individuals find dressing changes difficult — pain control is paramount. The limb is often hairless.

❖ **Poor pallor:** when the patient is lying flat in their bed, the poor pallor of their foot is an indication of ischaemia.

❖ **Dusky red or cyanotic blue appearance of the skin:** this occurs in some cases, where impaired perfusion has resulted in blood stagnation within dilated arterioles (Foster and Edmons, 1987).

Treatment

If an arterial ulcer is diagnosed, the individual should be immediately referred to a vascular surgeon. This is to determine if any surgical intervention can be carried out to improve perfusion and the blood supply to the limb. If surgery is not an option, due to the individual or their physical condition, conservative management is recommended. Where the wound requires dressing, it is generally felt that moist wound healing can predispose the individual to infection and healing will be compromised. This is due to poor perfusion and, therefore, the area is usually kept dry and infection free.

Mixed venous/arterial ulcers

These ulcers will have the features of a venous ulcer in combination with signs of arterial impairment (RCN, 1998)

A full lower leg assessment should be performed and if the ABPI is reduced (for example, <0.8), the patient should be referred for a routine vascular referral (RCN, 1998). To treat the venous component of the disease, and promote wound healing without causing further ischaemia or injury, use of reduced compression at levels of 23mmHg to 30mmHg is indicated if the ABPI is 0.6–0.8. The patient should be carefully monitored in these circumstances, paying particular attention to the correct application of compression to ensure that tissue injury does not occur (Bonham, 2003).

When carrying out assessments on the lower limb, the clinician should also consider the following co-morbidities during diagnosis.

Rheumatoid arthritis and systemic vasculitis

Individuals diagnosed with rheumatoid arthritis and systemic vasculitis are prone to leg ulceration. This is due to the skin over the tibial area being poorly vascularised. Trauma, or a vasculitic episode, can lead to the sudden occurrence of a lesion, which can deteriorate rapidly and be slow to heal. It is, however, generally recognised, that the aetiology of ulcers in patients with rheumatoid arthritis is not always clear (Cawley, 1987).

Vasculitic ulcers usually present as small, painful, multiple ulcers, with no indication of chronic venous hypertension. They are usually associated with inflammatory connective disorders such as polyarteritis nodosa and systemic lupus erythematosus (Morison and Moffat, 1994). Diagnosis can be difficult and specialist referral is recommended.

Due to the complex nature of the underlying disease processes, the healing of these wounds depends on the disease treatment and can be slow.

Table 2.3: Principles of management of leg ulcers

- All individuals with a leg ulcer should be assessed in line with national clinical guidelines

- A Doppler and/or LOI assessment of the circulation should be carried out by a skilled practitioner, and individuals with abnormal readings referred to a specialist

- Compression therapy remains the treatment of choice for venous leg ulceration

- Arterial leg ulceration should be referred for further vascular assessment. This is required to establish the extent of the occlusion and the presence of small vessel disease. A specialist assessment will determine whether the patient is suitable for angioplasty or major vascular surgery

- In mixed ulceration, features of venous ulcers in combination with signs of arterial impairment require assessment by an experienced practitioner. The person conducting the assessment should be aware that ulcers may be arterial, diabetic, rheumatoid or malignant, and refer the patient for specialist medical assessment (RCN, 1998). Reduced compression therapy should only be carried out by a competent practitioner

- Due to the complex nature of diabetic lower leg ulceration, it is advisable to obtain specialist referral by the multidisciplinary team and ensure a specialist Doppler assessment and the involvement of the diabetologist

---

Diabetes and neuropathy

Atherosclerosis is common in people with diabetes. It occurs bilaterally, and affects the microvascular as well as larger vessels. Individuals with long-term diabetes commonly suffer from sensory, motor, and autonomic neuropathy, due to impaired nerve function from hyperglycaemia. The combination of poor perfusion, altered sensation, and motor/nerve-induced foot deformity from neuropathy, results in limited joint mobility and gait alteration, which causes abnormal stress and pressure on the foot and leads to callus development. This increased pressure results in ulceration which, far too often in patients with diabetes, can cause infection, gangrene, and limb loss. Wound infection is particularly troublesome because it can occur without the individual's awareness of the usual signs of pain, swelling, and erythema, resulting in an extensive infection before it is recognised (Cooper et al, 2004).

Diabetic wounds

Diabetes is a common health condition. About 1.4 million people in the UK are known to have diabetes — that's about three in every 100 people. Diabetic foot ulcer management is complex in nature with a high rate of amputation. In a two-year retrospective study in Gwent, they had an amputation prevalence rate of 7% for diabetic patients (De et al, 2000). This has a huge psychosocial impact on the patient, as well as cost implications. Krentz et al (1997) estimated an annual hospital cost of £400,000 in a prospective survey conducted.

Diabetic foot wounds present as a significant clinical management challenge and carry high complication risks. Individuals with diabetic ulceration may have deceptively high pressure readings and, as such, should be referred for specialist assessment. Their ulcers are usually found on the foot, and often on bony prominences such as the bunion area or under the metatarsal heads, and they tend to be sloughy or necrotic in appearance (Cullum and Roe, 1995).

Patients with diabetes may have neuropathic, arterial and/or venous components (Browse et al, 1988; Nelzen et al, 1993). Consequently, all patients with diabetes with leg ulcers require a multidisciplinary approach to care, ensuring that the appropriate specialist referrals are made. It is essential that a diabetologist is involved in this process. Patients with type 2 diabetes have a three- to five-fold increased risk of developing peripheral arterial disease, compared to people without diabetes (Shearman and Chulakadabba, 1999; Hurst and Lee, 2003). For those individuals with peripheral arterial disease and diabetes, the risk of myocardial infarction and stroke are raised, and the rate of amputation is increased by as much as seven times (Dormandy and Murray, 1991).

Painful diabetic neuropathy symptoms are often slight at first. Some mild cases may go unnoticed for a long time. Numbness, pain, or tingling in the feet or legs may, after several years, lead to weakness in the muscles of the feet. Occasionally, diabetic neuropathy can flare up suddenly and affect specific nerves, and the patient will develop double vision or drooping eyelids, or weakness and atrophy of the thigh muscles. The loss of sensation in the feet may increase the possibility for foot injuries to go unnoticed and develop into ulcers or lesions that become infected.

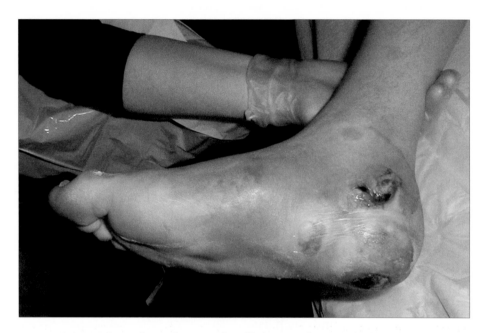

Figure 2.3: Diabetic foot ulcer, with cellulitis and osteomyelitis

Treatment

To ensure appropriate and effective treatment of this complex wound, the involvement of the whole multidisciplinary team is required. If the individual is experiencing pain, this should be addressed with an appropriate analgesic regime.

The wound should be assessed thoroughly, and any indication of infection should be eradicated with a topical antimicrobial and antibiotics (Benbow *et al*, 2004; Gray *et al*, 2003).

A full assessment should also determine the extent of the vascular/ nerve damage, and whether surgical intervention is required. The involvement of the podiatrist is essential to ensure correct shoeing and orthotic devices.

Table 2.4: Principles of management of diabetic wounds

- Diabetic foot wounds present a significant clinical management challenge and carry a high risk for those who suffer from them

- The two main features of foot ulceration are ischaemia and neuropathy, both of which predispose the individual to infection and lead to necrosis of the tissue

- Ensure the appropriate analgesia and antidepressants are prescribed for painful diabetic neuropathy (Benbow *et al*, 1999)

- Appropriate specialist referral should be made if the wound is infected

- Due to its complicated nature, a multidisciplinary approach to patient care is required when this problem manifests itself

Surgical wounds

There are many varied surgical techniques that can result in the development of a wound, such as:

- incisions or excisions
- investigative or corrective surgery
- open or keyhole surgery.

The following four types of wound healing are generally recognised (Thomas, 1990):

- primary closure, healing by first intention
- open granulation, healing by secondary intention
- delayed or secondary closure, sometimes called healing by third intention or tertiary intention
- grafting or flap formation.

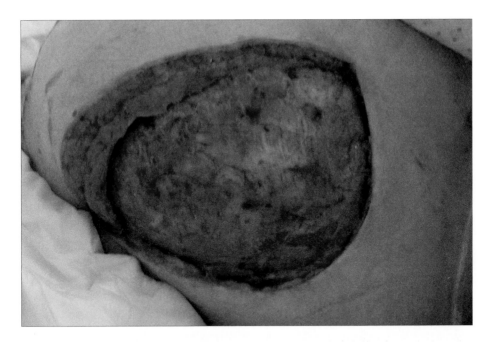

Figure 2.4: Surgical wound (abdominal cavity)

Healing by primary intention

Most clean surgical wounds are managed by primary closure. In this technique, the surgeon approximates the edges of the wound and individually sutures the different layers of tissue together. Primary closure is achieved by using either sutures, staples, Steri-Strips™ (3M™), tissue adhesives or a combination of all of these (Cooper _et al_, 2004). These wounds usually seal within twenty-four to forty-eight hours, and heal in eight to ten days when removal of sutures or staples takes place at the discretion of the surgeon. These wounds are usually covered in a low-adherent island dressing for the first twenty-four to forty-eight hours, and then are left exposed.

Healing by secondary intention

Secondary intention is often indicated in wounds that have sustained a degree of tissue loss as a result of surgery, or where an area has been excised and drained, due to abscess formation or pilonoidal sinus excision. Primary closure may be considered undesirable or impossible because of the extent of tissue loss, which makes it difficult to bring the edges of the wound together, or where pus may still be present, making the recurrence of infection high if primary closure were to be carried out. In these situations, the surgeon may favour leaving the wound open to heal by secondary intention. The duration of healing will vary in each individual case; wound healing is often affected by intrinsic and extrinsic factors that may result in complications (Baxter, 2003). As with all dressing choices, the primary function of a wound dressing is to promote healing by maintaining a moist wound environment. If healing by secondary intention, each dressing needs to be tailored to the size, depth, position and exudate level of the wound.

Healing by tertiary intention

Delayed primary closure is rather less commonly used. This occurs when the surgeon asserts that primary closure may be unsuccessful at the time of surgery, due to infection, poor blood supplies, or the need for excessive tension during closure. Patients will usually return for primary closure three to four days later. During this time, the dressing choice will be similar to that when left to heal by secondary intention.

Grafting or flap formation

A skin graft is an area of skin that is surgically removed from one part of the body and transplanted to another. The skin graft replaces tissue that has been destroyed, or creates new tissue where none exists. The major disadvantage of this technique is that another wound is created from the donor site. The most common types of skin grafts are partial-thickness or split skin grafts. These are removed from a suitable donor site, such as the thigh or buttock; donor sites usually heal rapidly within ten to fourteen days. Full-thickness skin grafts are used for more specialist surgery, where fat, hair, and sebaceous glands, are removed for transplanting.

Skin flaps usually involve epidermis, dermis, subcutaneous tissue and blood vessels. Flaps are selected when an area of full-thickness tissue loss occurs. The flap can be completely removed from the donor area and applied to a recipient area, where the blood vessels will be anastamosed to ensure viability of the flap — this can be referred to as a free island flap. Another method of flap is a rotational flap, where an area of tissue can be lifted and rotated to cover a defect which is in close proximity, but where the blood supply is still maintained.

Table 2.5: Principles of management of surgical wounds
• There are many varied surgical techniques that can result in the development of a wound: incisions or excisions, investigative or corrective, open or keyhole
• Four types of wound healing are generally recognised: primary closure, healing by first intention; open granulation, healing by secondary intention; delayed or secondary closure, sometimes called healing by third intention or tertiary intention; and grafting or flap formation
• The two main potential complications following surgical intervention are infection and dehiscence
• Early identification of surgical wound infection can reduce the damage to the wound
• The aim for all surgical wounds is to provide an optimal wound healing environment, which involves minimal disturbance to the wound and the prevention of bacterial invasion

Surgical wound complications

The two main complications following surgical intervention are infection and dehiscence. Early signs of wound infection are defined by redness, pain, heat and swelling of the wound and peri-wound area. These signs must not be confused with the inflammatory stage of wound healing, around days three to seven post-operatively.

Infection, among other contributing factors, can lead to dehiscence of the surgical wound: where the wound either partially or fully opens following primary closure. The options following dehiscence are to allow the wound to heal by secondary intention or by delayed closure.

Post-operative wound care will vary from centre to centre and practitioner to practitioner. However, the treatment aims for all surgical wounds are to provide an optimal wound healing environment, which involves minimal disturbance to the wound, and prevention of bacterial invasion.

Traumatic wounds

Skin tears

Skin tears usually occur in the elderly, or individuals with friable skin, and are often due to underlying medical conditions or long-term use of steroid medications. The trauma is frequently located in the individual's extremities, such as arms and lower leg, where an accidental bump or knock causes a skin tear and the epidermis is displaced but still retains the blood supply.

The most efficient way to manage these wounds is to reapply the skin tear, trying to bring the wound edges together to heal by first intention. This may be achieved by initially moistening the wound to facilitate reapplication of the skin tear. Once reapplied, Steri-Strips™ and/or a non-adhesive dressing can retain the skin tear; this should be secured using an appropriate secondary dressing.

If treated at the time of injury and the skin is reapplied, even with the most friable of skin, good skin cover can be achieved.

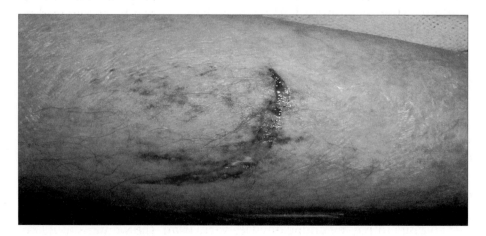

Figure 2.5: Skin tear

Grazes and abrasions

Grazes and abrasions are superficial injuries which are caused by falling onto a rough or gritty surface and the skin is rubbed or torn (Dealey, (1994). They should be cleansed thoroughly to ensure that no foreign bodies remain embedded in the wound bed. Due to the nature of their occurrence, these wounds are often painful.

The majority of these wounds can be effectively treated with a simple, non/low-adherent dressing. However, if painful, the individual may benefit from the application of a film or hydrocolloid dressing, which occludes the wound and keeps the nerve endings moist, therefore reducing the pain. Due to their superficial nature, these wounds should heal quite quickly.

Lacerations

A laceration is a wound caused by blunt trauma, which has split or torn the skin forming jagged wound edges (Collins _et al_, 2002). A thorough assessment of the wound should be carried out to ensure that there is no underlying structure trauma. If the wound edges are clean, closure can be obtained by first intention through Steri-Strips™, glue, or suturing (Dealey, 1994). If the wound is contaminated, primary closure is not indicated, and the wound should be treated with a topical antimicrobial until the infection is cleared. The wound should then be encouraged to heal by secondary intention and moist wound management.

Penetrating and stab wounds

Knives, bullets or other sharp missiles may cause penetrating wounds (Thomas, 1990). Although the external appearance of a penetrating wound may suggest that the injury is relatively minor, internal damage can be considerable, depending upon the site and depth of the penetration, and/or the velocity of the bullet or missile (Owen-Smith, 1985). Prior to implementing any treatment plan, the wound should be thoroughly explored by a doctor as surgery may be necessary.

Table 2.6: Principles of management of traumatic wounds

- Identify and, if appropriate, remove the source of trauma

- If the wound is contaminated or debris is present, ensure that it is cleansed thoroughly

- Thorough assessment should be carried out to ascertain if there is any underlying structure trauma

- Treat the wound following the principles of the Wound Healing Continuum, based on accurate classification and wound assessment

- Always document plan of care and action taken in the individual's care records

Burns

Burns require separate consideration from other traumatic wounds, due to the specialised nature of care required for their treatment. The following show the varying forms of burns.

- **Thermal burns:** these can either be caused by dry heat, such as fires, flash flames, friction, or by wet heat, usually referred to as scalds from hot liquid.

- **Chemical burns:** these involve chemicals of an acid or alkaline nature.

- **Electrical burns:** these can be low voltage, usually a domestic accident <1,000 volts. High voltage burns are industrial accidents, often involving power lines, >1,000 volts.

- **Radiation burns:** these are caused by accidental exposure to ultra-violet light, x-rays and gamma rays.

Extent of burns

The extent of a burn is described by a percentage that indicates the amount of the total body surface area (TBSA) involved. There is little consensus to determine what constitutes a minor scald, which can be treated as an outpatient, and what TBSA should be involved before a referral to a specialist centre is made (Fowler, 1999). Young patients with 5%–10% TBSA should be referred to a specialist centre along with adults who have 5%–10% burns to their face and hands (Turner, 1998). Any individual with 10% or more of the TBSA as a superficial partial-thickness burn would benefit from a review at a specialist centre.

Burn classifications

The depth of tissue penetrated by the thermal insult determines the classification of the burn. The various levels of severity are:

* **Superficial burns:** these only involve the epidermis. The skin is dry and intact, but very red and painful to touch. They may form blisters but will usually heal within three to seven days, with minimal or no treatment depending on the formation of the blister (Fowler, 1999). If the skin is intact, it may help to apply a bland moisturiser, or after-sun, to keep the skin supple and rehydrated.

* **Superficial partial-thickness burns:** these involve the epidermis and the superficial layer of the dermis. The skin usually shows immediate blistering, is moist and exudes haemoserous fluid. These burns are very painful for the individual (Fowler, 1999). Treatment will require debridement of the blistered areas using a conservative sharp debridement technique. If the wound was contaminated at time of injury, treatment with a topical antimicrobial would be recommended to prevent complications from infection. If the wound is clean, limit dressing changes by applying an absorbent non-adherent dressing, but also ensure that it does not incapacitate the individual's ability to move and exercise the affected area.

* **Deep partial-thickness, deep dermal burns:** these are burns which involve the epidermis and dermis, but leave the hair follicles and sebaceous glands intact (Fowler, 1999). The burn appears as white/creamy in colour, with blistering. They can be treated by either debridement and grafting, or, if the area is small, autolytic debridement of the burn tissue, and active treatment with moist dressings.

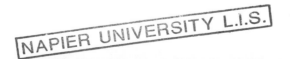

❖ **Full-thickness burns**: these involve all structural layers: epidermis, dermis, subcutaneous layer and/or deeper structures. The appearance of the skin is one of a waxy-white, grey area or yellow/black translucent leathery appearance (Fowler, 1999). Due to the damage of the nerve endings there is little pain associated with these wounds, but wound edges can be sensitive. These wounds require surgical intervention with extensive debridement and grafting.

Complex wounds

The title complex wounds refers to wounds which may have an underlying pathophysiology, eg. *pyoderma gangrenosum*, necrotising fasciitis, or where wounds may be complicated by the individual's prevalent medical condition, such as rheumatoid arthritis. It is beyond the scope of this chapter to discuss all of these types of wounds, however, the following will be discussed:

- *pyoderma gangrenosum*
- necrotising fasciitis
- fungating tumours.

Pyoderma gangrenosum

Pyoderma gangrenosum is an immunologically-mediated chronic necrotising ulcerative cutaneous condition of the skin (Powell and Perry, 1996). *Pyoderma gangrenosum* often affects a person with an underlying internal disease such as:

- inflammatory bowel diseases (ulcerative colitis and Crohn's disease)
- rheumatoid arthritis
- chronic active hepatitis
- tumours (solid) (Gudi *et al*, 2000).

Pyoderma gangrenosum usually starts quite suddenly, often at the site of a minor injury, and mainly affects the legs and feet (von den Driesch,

1997). It may start as a small pustule, red bump, or blood-blister. The skin then breaks down resulting in an ulcer. The ulcer can deepen and widen rapidly. Characteristically, the edge of the ulcer is purple and undermined as it enlarges. It is usually very painful. Several ulcers may develop at the same time. Left untreated, the ulcers may continue to enlarge, persist unchanged, or may slowly heal.

Treatment with oral or topical steroids is usually successful in arresting the process, but complete healing may take months. Modern moist wound healing products may play a role in promoting healing if the individual is commenced on oral steroids. Patients with *pyoderma gangrenosum* are normally cared for by a dermatologist.

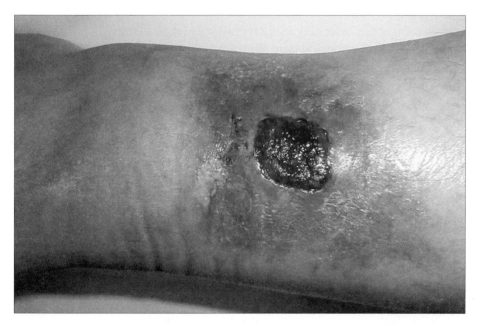

Figure 2.6: *Pyoderma gangrenosum*

Necrotising fasciitis

Necrotising fasciitis is a relatively rare, life-threatening condition, where bacterial toxins invade and destroy large areas of tissue. The most common bacteria associated with necrotising fasciitis is the group A haemolytic streptoccous, commonly known as *Streptococcus pyogenes*. It may enter the body through a long-standing chronic wound, or through an acute wound entry site (Timmons, 2005). Diagnosis can be difficult. The following clinical features are linked with necrotising fasciitis:

- rapid progression
- poor therapeutic response
- blistering necrosis
- cyanosis
- localised tenderness
- pyrexia
- tachycardia
- hypotension
- altered level of consciousness.

In cases of acute infection of previously unbroken skin, the time from injury to development of severe symptoms can be very short (0–2 hours).

Clinically, it often starts with pain — this may be increased pain if the wound already exists. The pain then changes to swelling and soft tissue erythema that does not respond to antibiotics. There is a rapid progression to a grey/blue skin followed by necrosis (Timmons, 2005).

Treatment

Intravenous antibiotics should be administered as soon as possible in an attempt to slow down the invading bacteria.

Aggressive surgical debridement is essential, with the removal of all non-viable tissue with a wide margin. This is to try and prevent recurrence.

Fungating tumours

Fungating wounds arise as the tumour infiltrates the skin and its supporting blood and lymphatic vessels. Unless the malignant cells are checked, the fungation extends and has the potential to cause massive damage to the wound through a combination of rapid growth, loss of vascularity, and ulceration and necrosis (Grocott, 2000).

The management of these wounds is complex, based on a balance between symptom control and patient comfort and acceptability. A great many decisions are reached as a result of information provided by the individual; what they are experiencing and their concerns. Issues relating to pain, odour and exudate are frequently raised, and these should be prioritised when assessing and implementing care.

Table 2.7: Principles of management of complex wounds
• Rapid diagnosis and specialist referral
• Always establish the underlying pathology of the wound
• Recognise the impact that underlying conditions such as rheumatoid arthritis might have
• Seek specialist advice or referral to ensure that the underlying pathology is managed effectively

These types of wound are an example of where an underlying condition can result in the development of a wound: emphasising the need to identify the factors that have led to the development of the wound. Where a wound cannot be identified as fitting into the first five categories, it can be categorised as a complex wound and consideration should be given to the need for specialist referral/advice. Wounds, such as fungating lesions, vasculitic ulcers, or those of unknown pathology, are other examples of complex wounds.

Conclusion

The management of wounds is based on an understanding of the wound's aetiology, any underlying pathophysiology, a full assessment and then appropriate treatment interventions. This chapter provides an overview of some of the common wound types and highlights their key management principles.

References

Allman RM (1997) Pressure ulcer prevalence, incidence, risk factors and impact. *Clin Geriatric Med* **13**(3): 421–36

Baxter H (2003) Management of surgical wounds. *Nurs Times* **99**(13): 66–8

Benbow SJ, Cossins L, MacFarlane IA (1999) Painful diabetic neuropathy. *Diabetic Med* **16**: 632–44

Benbow SJ, Daousi C, MacFarlane IA (2004) Diagnosing and managing chronic painful diabetic neuropathy. *The Diabetic Foot* **7**(1): 34–44

Berg RW (1986) Etiology and pathophysiology of diameter dermatitis. *Adv Dermatol* **3**: 102–6

Bliss M (1990) (Editorial) Preventing pressure sores. *Lancet* **335**: 1311–12

Bianchi J (2005) LOI: an alternative to Doppler in leg ulcer patients. *Wounds UK* **1**(1): 80–5

Bonham P (2003) Assessment and management of patients with venous, arterial, and diabetic/neuropathic lower extremity wounds. *Am Association of Critical Care Nurses* **14**(4): 442–56

Browse NL, Burns KG, Lea Thomas M (1988) *Diseases of the Veins: pathology, diagnosis and treatment.* Edward Arnold, London

Cawley MI (1987) Vasculitis and ulceration in rheumatic diseases of the foot. *Baillieres Clin Rheumatol* **1**(2): 315–33

Cullum N, Roe B (1995) *Leg Ulcers Nursing Management — a reasearch-based guide.* Baillière Tindall, London

Cooper P, Russell F, Stringfellow SA (2004) A review of different wound types and their principles of management. *Applied Wound Management Supplement I.* Wounds UK, Aberdeen

Cornwall J, Dore CJ, Lewis JD (1986) Leg ulcers: epidemiology and aetiology. *Br J Surg* **73**: 693–6

Dormandy JA, Murray GD (1991) The fate of the claudicant: a prospective study of 1969 claudicants. *Eur J Vasc Surg* **5**: 131–3

Dealey C (1994) *The Care of Wounds.* Blackwell Science, Oxford

De P, Kunze G, Gibby OM, Harding K (2000) Outcome of diabetic foot ulcers in a specialist foot clinic. *The Diabetic Foot* **4**(3): 131–6

Defloor T, Grypdonck MHF (1999) Sitting posture and prevention of pressure ulcers. *Applied Nursing Research* **12**(3): 136–42

European Pressure Ulcer Advisory Panel (2002) Guide to pressure ulcer grading. *EPUAP Review* **3**(3): 75

Fiers SA (1996) Breaking the cycle: The etiology of incontinence dermatitis and evaluating and using skin care products. *Ostomy Wound Management* **42**(3): 33–43

Foster A, Edmons ME (1987) Examination of the diabetic foot. *Practical Diabetes* 4(3): 105–6

Fowler A (1999) Burns. In: Miller M, Glover D, eds. *Wound Management Theory and Practice*. Nursing Times Books, London

Gebhardt K, Bliss MR (1994) Preventing pressure sores in orthopedic patients — is prolonged chair nursing detrimental? *J Tissue Viability* 4(2): 51–4

Gosnell D (1973) An assessment tool to identify pressure sores. *Nurs Residential Care* 22: 55–9

Gray D, White RJ, Cooper P (2003) The wound healing continuum. In: White RJ, ed. *The Silver Book*. Quay Books, MA Healthcare Ltd, London

Gray D, Cooper P, Clark M (1999) Pressure ulcer prevention in an acute hospital. Poster presentation EPUAP, Amsterdam 1999

Grocott P (2000) The palliative management of fungating malignant wounds. *J Wound Care* 9(1): 4–9

Gudi VS, Julian C, Bowers PW (2000) Pyoderma gangrenosum complicating bilateral mammoplasty. *Br J Plastic Surg* 53: 440–1

Günnewicht B, Dunford C (2004) *Fundamental Aspects of Tissue Viability Nursing*. Quay Books, MA Healthcare Ltd, London

Hurst RT, Lee RW (2003) Increased incidence of coronary artherosclerosis in type 2 diabetes mellitus: mechanisms and management. *Ann Intern Med* 139: 824–34

Jones J (2000) The use of holistic assessment in the treatment of leg ulcers. *Br J Nurs* 9(16): 1040–52

Jordan MM, Clark M, Barbanel CL *et al* (1977) Incidence of pressure sores in the Greater Glasgow health Board area. *Lancet* 2: 548–50

Leyden JJ, Katz S, Stewart R, Kligman AM (1977) Urinary ammonia and ammonia producing micro-organisms in infants with and without diaper dermatitis. *Arch Dermatol* 113: 1678–80

Krentz AM, Acheson P, Basu A, Kilvert A, Wright AD, Nattrass M (1997) Morbidity and mortality associated with diabetic foot disease: a 12-month prospective survey of hospital admissions in a single UK centre. *Foot* 7: 144–7

Maklebust J (1987) Pressure ulcers, aetiology and prevention. *Nurs Clin North Am* 22(2): 359–77

Morison M, Moffat C (1994) *A Colour Guide to the Assessment and Management of Leg Ulcers*. Mosby, St Louis

Nelzen O, Bergqvist D, Lindhagen A (1993) High prevalence of diabetes in chronic leg ulcer patients: a cross-sectional population study. *Diabet Med* 10: 345–50

NHS Quality Improvement (2003) *Best Practice Statement for the Prevention of Pressure Ulcers*. NHS Quality Improvement, Scotland

Norton D, McLaren R, Exton-Smith A (1962) *An Investigation of Geriatric Nursing Problems in Hospital*. Churchill, Livingstone, Edinburgh

Owen-Smith M (1985) Wounds caused by the weapons of war. In: Westaby S, ed. *Wound Care*. Heinemann Medical, London: 110–20

Powell FC, Su WP, Perry HO (1996) Pyoderma gangrenosum: classification and management. *J Am Acad Dertmatol* **34**: 395–409

Pudner R (1998) The management of patients with a leg ulcer. *J Community Nurs* **12**(5): 26–33

Royal College of Nursing (1998) *Clinical Practice Guidelines: The Management of Patients with Venous Leg Ulcers*. RCN Institute, Centre for Evidence-Based Nursing, University of York and the School of Nursing, Midwifery and Health Visiting, University of Manchester

Rycroft-Malone J (2000) *Clinical Practice Guidelines. Pressure Ulcer Risk Assessment and Prevention*. RCN, London

Scottish Intercollegiate Guidelines Network (1998) *The Care of Patients with Chronic Leg Ulcers*. SIGN, Edinburgh

Shearman CP, Chulakadabba A (1999) The value of risk factor management in patients with peripheral arterial disease. In: *The Evidence for Vascular Surgery*. Tfm Publishing, Harley, Shropshire

Sumner DS (1989) Non-invasive assessment of peripheral arterial occlusive disease. In: Rutherford KS, ed. *Vascular Surgery*. 3rd edn. WB Saunders, Philadelphia

Thomas S (1990) *Wound Management and Dressings*. The Pharmaceutical Press, London

Timmons J (2005) Recognising fasciitis. *Wounds UK* **1**(2): 40–5

Torrance C (1983) *Pressure Sore: Aetiology, treatment and prevention*. Croom Helm, London

Towey AP, Erland SM (1988) Validity and reliability of an assessment tool for pressure ulcer risk. *Decubitus* **1**(2): 40–2

Turner DG (1998) Ambulatory care of the burn patient. In: Carrougher GJ, ed. *Burn Care and Therapy*. Mosby, St Louis

Von den Driech P (1997) Pyoderma gangrenosum: a report of 44 cases with follow-up. *Br J Dermatol* **137**: 1000–5

Waterlow J (1985) A risk assessment card. *Nurs Times* **81**(48): 49–55

Wounds UK (2005) *Best Practice Statement for Compression Hosiery*. Wounds UK, Aberdeen

Young T (2004) The 30-degree tilt vs the 90-degree lateral and supine positions in reducing the incidence of non-blanching erythema in a hospital inpatient population: a randomised controlled trial. *J Tissue Viability* **14**(3): 88, 90, 92–6

CHAPTER 3

APPLIED WOUND MANAGEMENT

David Gray, Richard White, Pam Cooper, Andrew Kingsley

Part I: Introduction

Wound management is a constantly evolving speciality, with regular developments in terms of products and knowledge. The assessment of wounds is a subjective matter, with methods varying considerably from one clinician to another (Fletcher, 2003). Uniformity and consistency in assessment are key to continuity of quality care; hence, a standard for assessment is essential. In recent years, many systems of wound assessment have been published, each focusing on the type of tissues in the wound as a basic assessment parameter. The practical use of such an approach is intended to add consistency in management from clinician to clinician, and to provide a quick reference to the progress in healing. The most recent advances have seen the introduction of Applied Wound Management (AWM; Gray *et al*, 2005), Wound Bed Preparation (WBP; Schultz *et al*, 2003; Jones, 2004) and TIME (Dowsett and Ayello, 2004), concepts which clearly promote the adoption of systematic approaches to wound management. The key principles underlying the concepts (debridement, wound bioburden control, and exudate management), have been recognised as good practice for some time (Dealey, 1994; Sibbald *et al*, 2000).

Within the UK, little is known of the true extent of wound healing by secondary intention. National average healing rates for leg ulcers and pressure ulcers simply do not yet exist: in fact, it is very difficult to even estimate how many of these wounds exist in the first place. The AWM framework allows the categorisation of most wounds healing by secondary intention and, if applied in a clinical setting, can facilitate clinical audit, producing data which could define the true extent of wounds healing by secondary intention in the UK.

This chapter presents the Applied Wound Management (AWM) framework that utilises three different continuums, each relating to a key wound parameter:

❖ **Wound Healing Continuum (WHC):** is represented by the tissues in the wound and is a colour-based continuum.

❖ **Wound Infection Continuum (WIC):** is subdivided into named stages representing varying host responses to bioburden, each identified by clinical cues.

❖ **Wound Exudate Continuum (WEC):** is represented by volume and consistency parameters, and each can be graded according to a 'matrix' continuum.

This practical application to everyday wound care will enable the practitioner to approach wound assessment logically and systematically. Increased workloads across the NHS require decision-making to be systematic, clear and coherent. The AWM system aids this type of decision-making, reducing the risk of poor practice and litigation.

Part II: Using the Wound Healing Continuum to assess tissue

While practitioners may be looking at the same wound, they often articulate what they see in different ways (Dealey, 1994). The Wound Healing Continuum (Gray *et al*, 2003) is a system designed to introduce essential consistency into wound assessment and wound description.

Wound tissue types

The tissues in a wound (within the wound bed and margins), if left to heal by secondary intention, indicate the relevant pathologies present, reflect the state of healing and, consequently, the success of the management approach. Thus, a black wound (as opposed to black skin changes in melanoma, gangrene or frostbite) indicates the presence of eschar or necrosis (Bale, 1997). Wound eschar is full-thickness, dry, devitalised (dead) tissue that has arisen through prolonged local ischaemia. In relation to pressure ulcers, eschar might arise after a sudden large vessel occlusion caused by a shearing injury (Witkowski and Parish, 1982). Unless removed, the eschar will delay healing, as healing cannot proceed effectively without a moist wound environment (Winter, 1962; Parnham, 2002).

Wound tissue that is yellow and fibrous, adheres to the wound bed, and cannot be removed on irrigation, indicating the presence of slough (Tong, 1999). This adherent, fibrous material is derived from the proteins fibrin and fibrinogen (Tong, 1999). In combination with wound exudate, it serves as an ideal environment for bacterial growth and, consequently, infection (Colebrook *et al*, 1960; O'Brien, 2002; Davies, 2004). It also serves to impair healing by restricting re-epithelialisation (Kubo *et al*, 2001). The clinical objective of managing a sloughy wound is to debride (Tong, 1999; Hampton, 2005).

The red, moist tissue in a wound is a combination of new blood vessel growth (angiogenesis), and a matrix of fibroblasts (connective tissue or dermal cells) known as granulation tissue. This is usually indicative of a healing wound and is often accompanied by signs of re-epithelialisation (epidermal regrowth) (Gray *et al*, 2003). It is important to remember that not all red wounds are healthy; they may be critically colonised and non-healing/static, or show evidence of haemolytic bacteria (if a dull brick-red colour) (Dowsett *et al*, 2004).

Colour and wound assessment

Previous assessment methods have used wound colour as the basis for identifying the tissues of clinical importance. For ease of identification, necrosis is termed 'black', slough 'yellow', granulation 'red', and epithelialisation 'pink'. The earliest colour systems were based on three colours: red, black and yellow (Cuzzell, 1988, 1995; Stotts, 1990; Loughry, 1991; Krasner, 1995; Meaume *et al*, 1997; Lorentzen *et al*, 1999; de Peyrolle, 2002). This approach has been described as being easy to use and to teach (Goldman and Salcido, 2002), but is criticised for being simplistic (Maklebust, 1997). In some instances, the inclusion of green, to signify infection (wounds containing *Pseudomonas aeruginosa* are often green or green-blue) has been used. This is also too simplistic as there is no evidence to suggest that a green or green-blue wound is infected, ie. anything other than colonised or critically colonised (Davis, 1998; Kingsley, 2003; Villavicenzio, 1998).

The approach taken in the Wound Healing Continuum is to incorporate intermediate colour combinations between the four key colours (*Figure 3.1*).

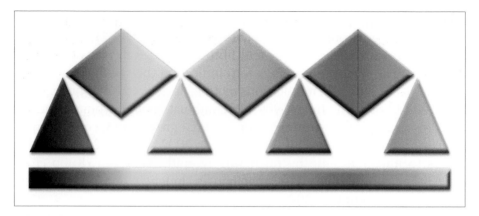

Figure 3.1: The Wound Healing Continuum

To use this system to the optimum clinical benefit, it is first important to identify the colour that is furthest to the left of the continuum. For example, if the wound contains yellow slough and red granulation tissue, it would be defined as a 'yellow/red wound'. A key objective of the consequent wound management plan would be to remove the yellow tissue and promote the growth of red granulation tissue (Gray *et al*, 2005). In this instance, the management plan should focus on removal of the yellow sloughy tissue, and promotion of the red granulation tissue. As this objective is achieved, the wound can progress along the continuum towards the right to the 'pink /healing' status. It is important to remember that, in addition to this focus on the wound bed and margins, care must be taken to protect the skin surrounding the wound. The interaction of otherwise healthy skin with exudate can lead to maceration and wound enlargement (White and Cutting, 2003).

Identifying and obtaining treatment objectives

Debridement

Where the wound exhibits dead tissue, eg. black, black/yellow, yellow, or yellow/red, a key treatment aim should be the debridement of the devitalised tissue unless contraindicated by the patient's overall physical condition or disease process, such as peripheral vascular disease (PVD) (European Tissue Repair Society [ETRS], 2003). There are a large number of debridement options open to the practitioner, and each patient's requirements are unique and require individual management. Many different clinical presentations and challenges are likely to face the practitioner when a wound needs to be debrided. The volume and viscosity of exudate present, or the presence of infection, must be considered, but the types of treatment available can be categorised into three separate categories:

- active
- autolytic (moisture donation)
- autolytic (moisture absorption).

Active debridement

❖ **Surgical debridement:** Surgical debridement involves removal of dead tissue from the wound bed. It is usually carried out under surgical conditions in locations such as operating theatres, and results in a bleeding wound bed. This form of debridement is carried out by surgeons/podiatrists and specialist nurses, using surgical instruments such as scalpels and forceps. Surgical debridement removes dead tissue and results in an inflammatory response from the wound, thus stimulating healing (Bale, 1997).

❖ **Sharp debridement:** Sharp debridement is the removal of dead tissue. This technique involves debulking the wound of slough and necrotic tissue (ie. reducing the amount of dead tissue within the wound). As the objective is not to create a bleeding wound bed (that is the complete removal of dead tissue), some slough and necrosis is left. The removal of dead tissue, as may be achieved by sharp debridement, is essential for wound healing (O'Brien, 2002). This process, unlike surgical debridement, is usually carried out at the patient's bedside, or in the patient's own home. It requires the use of surgical instruments, such as a specialist wound debridement pack.

❖ **Larval therapy:** The use of maggot larvae to debride the wound of dead tissue has become a mainstream therapy in the UK during the past decade. The larvae liquefy the dead tissue and, where the treatment is successful, can result in rapid debridement (Thomas *et al*, 1998).

Autolytic debridement

Autolytic debridement is the process by which the body attempts to shed devitalised tissue by the use of moisture. Where tissue can be kept moist it will naturally degrade and deslough from the underlying healthy structures. This process is facilitated by the presence of enzymes (matrix metalloproteinases) which disrupt the proteins that bind the dead tissue to the body (Schultz *et al*, 2003). The process can be enhanced by the application of wound management products which promote a moist environment. These products can be divided into two categories: those that donate moisture to the dead tissue, and those that absorb excess moisture produced by the body. Both are designed to facilitate the autolytic debridement process.

❖ **Autolytic (moisture donation):** The group of products listed in *Figure* 3.2 facilitate autolytic debridement by donating moisture to the dead tissue, and are designed to facilitate the natural process of autolysis. Hydrocolloids, hydrogels, honey and silver sulphadiazine donate moisture to the wound and thus enhance the process of debridement (Cooper *et al*, 2003). These products can be used at all stages of the Wound Healing Continuum, and some also have antimicrobial activity. The use of antimicrobial products should always be based on clinical need and not used as a matter of routine.

❖ **Autolytic (moisture absorption):** The groups of products listed in *Figure* 3.2 (alginates, cadexomer iodine and Hydrofiber®) facilitate autolytic debridement by absorbing moisture from the wound (exudate) while ensuring that the necrotic tissue does not dry out (Cooper *et al*, 2003). By absorbing excess exudate, these products avoid damage to the surrounding skin from maceration. As with the moisture-donating products, some of the products within the moisture-absorption group also have an antimicrobial effect. *Figure* 3.2 indicates where these products can be used across the Wound Healing Continuum.

Treatment options		Black	Black/Yellow	Yellow	Yellow/Red	Red	Red/Pink	Pink
Active								
	Surgical debridement							
	Sharp debridement							
	Larval therapy							
Autolytic [Moisture donation]								
	Hydrocolloids							
	Hydrogels							
	Honey #							
	Silver sulphadiazine #							
Autolytic [Moisture absorption]								
	Alginates *							
	Cadexomer iodine #							
	Hydrofiber® *							

Figure 3.2: Wound management treatment: debridement
These products have an antimicrobial effect
* Some products in this category have antimicrobial effects

Clinical use of debridement techniques

It is likely that during the debridement process, treatments from more than one group may be required to achieve full debridement of the wound. The heel pressure ulcer presented in *Figure 3.3*, shows necrotic tissue which has been rehydrated using an autolytic (moisture-donating) treatment. As a result of donating moisture to the necrotic tissue, the necrotic eschar has begun to lift at the wound margins, separating from the slough below. The necrotic tissue is categorised as 'black' on the Wound Healing Continuum.

In *Figure 3.4*, the wound has been subjected to sharp debridement and the necrotic tissue removed to leave the slough below exposed. The wound is now categorised as a 'yellow' wound on the Wound Healing Continuum. No bleeding or pain has been caused. Following sharp debridement, the patient is treated with a moisture-donating product to continue the process of autolytic debridement.

The wound in *Figure 3.5* is producing high levels of moisture which need to be absorbed. The wound bed is covered with slough which requires debriding. The wound is categorised as a 'yellow/red' wound on the Wound Healing Continuum. By utilising an autolytic (moisture-absorption) treatment, the wound is successfully debrided and has moved on to the next stage of the Healing Continuum — 'red' (*Figure 3.6*).

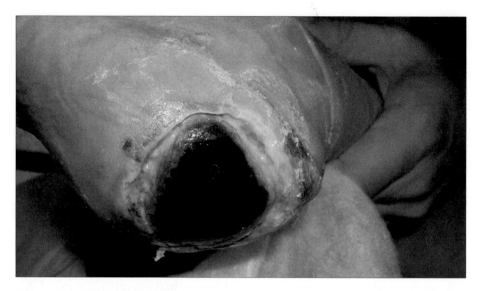

Figure 3.3: Black wound

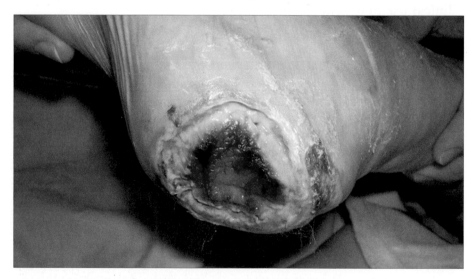

Figure 3.4: Black/yellow wound post-sharp debridement

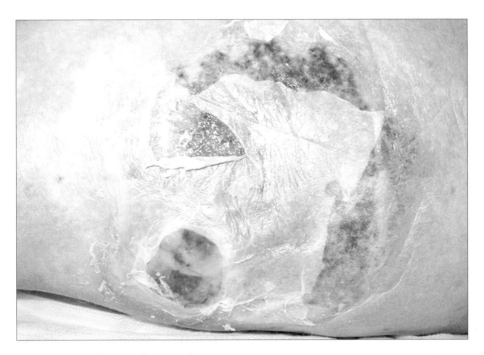

Figure 3.5: Yellow/red wound

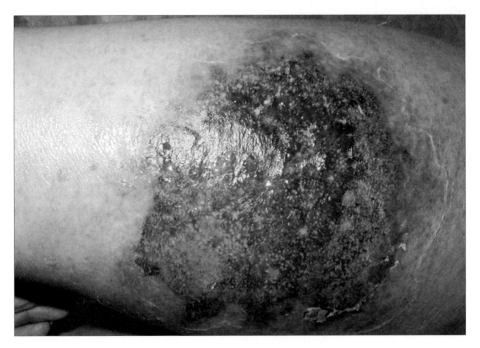

Figure 3.6: Red wound

Granulation and epithelialisation

Granulation (red) and epithelial (pink) tissue are the final two stages of the Wound Healing Continuum. Granulation tissue is formed in the wound bed as a result of the action of fibroblasts stimulated by the growth factors provided by macrophages. Angiogenesis, the development of new capillary buds, leads to the development of new blood vessels. Granulation presents as a red, uneven surface. It is highly vascular and needs to be kept moist to facilitate its growth. As granulation develops in the wound, the margins begin to show signs of epithelial growth and pink tissue forms across the surface of the granulation tissue. This is the final stage of healing. This layer is only one cell thick and requires protection from desiccation and trauma. Where a wound has been categorised as 'red' or 'red/pink', the main objective is the promotion of granulation tissue and then epithelialisation.

Both granulation and epithelial tissue need to be kept moist and protected from trauma. There are three different categories of treatment available when healing by secondary intention: active, moisture donation and moisture absorption. Many products can either donate or absorb moisture in a granulating wound and, for the purposes of this chapter, they have been categorised in relation to their main function as interpreted by the authors. Some active treatments, such as skin grafting and skin substitutes, have not been included in this chapter.

Active treatment

Topical negative pressure therapy (VAC — vacuum assisted closure) is used in the management of large granulating wounds, particularly cavity wounds. It works by placing a foam pad into the wound, which is then sealed and negative pressure applied via a vacuum pump. This facilitates the promotion of granulation tissue, as well as removing excess exudate (Moore, 2005). As a result of the partial vacuum created by the therapy, exudate is removed from the wound while still maintaining a moist wound environment (Banwell, 1999). Where high exudate levels occur, such as in severe pressure ulcers or dehisced abdominal wounds, this therapy can facilitate the management of large volumes of exudate. Angiogenesis can be stimulated by the application of topical negative pressure (Argenta and Morykwas, 1997).

Moisture donation

The fragile nature of granulation tissue means that it has to be kept moist to prevent desiccation and delayed tissue growth. Products, such as hydrocolloids, hydrogels and honey, can all deliver moisture to the wound bed, thus supporting granulation. Hydrocolloids, sheet hydrogels and sheet honey dressings can also provide an element of moisture absorption (Cooper, *et al*, 2003), but this is not their main function, which is that of moisture donation. Some of these products may also have an antimicrobial action.

Moisture absorption

An excess of moisture on the wound bed can lead to maceration of the wound margins and delayed healing (Cameron and Powell, 1992). The products listed in *Figure 3.2* (alginates, cadexomer iodine, collagen products, foams and Hydrofiber®) absorb exudate, providing the ideal environment for the promotion of granulation tissue and epithelialisation of the wound. Some of the products may have an antimicrobial capability.

Promotion of granulation and epithelial tissue in clinical practice

In *Figure 3.7*, the patient has presented with an abrasion to the knee and the wound is categorised 'red' on the Wound Healing Continuum. An accurate assessment of the patient would reveal whether or not the wound is producing sufficient exudate to facilitate healing. Depending on the outcome of the assessment, the correct product selection will lead to a 'pink' wound as seen in *Figure 3.8*.

Conclusion

The Wound Healing Continuum supports a systematic assessment of the wound and the identification of clear treatment objectives. Where there is dead tissue, debridement is likely to be the treatment objective unless otherwise contraindicated by the patient's condition. Where debridement is identified as the treatment objective, the clinical judgement of the practitioner will be needed to decide the method of debridement required. As stated, it is likely that more than one method will be used as the wound progresses to a 'red' wound bed. It is important that treatments are prescribed only after a holistic assessment of the patient's needs has been carried out.

Similarly, following a systematic assessment of wounds in the 'yellow/red' to 'pink' categories, the treatments must be selected to promote granulation and meet the needs of the patient. Ensuring the rapid growth of granulation and epithelial tissue, not only reduces the time required to achieve healing, but also reduces the risk of wound infection (Gray *et al*, 2003). A balanced, moist environment can be achieved using many different treatments; however, it is vital that the selection of such treatments is underpinned by regular, accurate assessments.

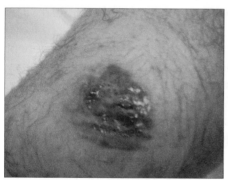

Figure 3.7: Red wound

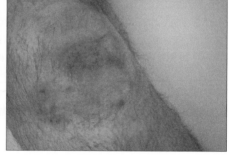

Figure 3.8: Pink wound

Part III: Using the Wound Infection Continuum to assess wound bioburden

From a clinical management perspective, it is the recognition of the state of the wound – with respect to the infection status – that is the challenge. Research informs us of the bacteria that contribute to the wound bioburden and of the criteria for infection. However, the key to good wound management is to avoid infection. Thus, it becomes important to recognise the subtle signs and symptoms that precede infection, and to intervene accordingly. These factors are included in the evolving 'Wound Infection Continuum' and the related treatment guidelines.

Wound bioburden: a factor for chronicity

Many wounds healing by secondary intention become indolent, causing extended periods of discomfort and inconvenience for the patient, as well as an increase in healthcare costs and workload for staff. A common cause for this indolence is the effect of the wound bioburden (Browne *et al*, 2001); this is the result of either invasive infection, the quantity or mixture of microbes present, or, the effect of their various virulence determinants (ie. toxins; Finlay and Falkow, 1997). The indiscriminate use of antibiotics in all open wounds will raise healthcare costs and contribute to the development and selection of multi-resistant micro-organisms. Therefore, systemic antibiotics are reserved for proven cases of spreading wound infection.

However, diagnosis of infection is restricted to the recognition of certain clinical signs and symptoms, with qualitative microbiology providing information for the checking of empirically-initiated antibiotic prescriptions for the identified species and strain-resistant patterns they possess. The use of microbiology (qualitative, semi-quantitative or quantitative) alone, is flawed, because results require interpretation based on the prevailing wisdom of the relative importance of bacteria and/or quantities of bacteria, in any particular context, on the body. As infection is a clinical diagnosis, there remains large scope for either over- or under-treatment, dependent on the diagnostic skills of the clinician.

Wounds that do not exhibit the classical signs of infection may become indolent through the effects of bioburden and, although they might benefit from an antimicrobial strategy, either topical or systemic, they often go untreated. Improving the clinician's ability to make a clinical diagnosis requires a consolidation of microbiological status, and the incorporation of clinical signs and symptoms into an easily understood package. It could be argued that there is no clear consensus as to what constitutes the clinical signs of wound infection; however, these have recently been clarified (Cutting and White, 2005; EWMA, 2005).

Thus, it is necessary to extrapolate the principles of microbiological growth, transmission and pathological potential developed in the laboratory to the clinical setting. The concept for building a bridge between microbiological theory and clinical practice is called the Wound Infection Continuum. This continuum seeks, in a simplified form, to align the states of colonisation, critical colonisation, local infection and spreading infection, with the probable bacterial bioburden and host response, enabling the practitioner to interpret what is happening. In clinical practice, the main focus is on reducing the high levels of organisms that are causing problems. However, the ultimate aim is to achieve this without toxicity to healing cells, bacterial resistance, or elevating costs.

The continuum uses conceptual names for increasingly severe forms of wound bioburden that link with the patient's host (immune) response. The use of the term 'continuum' in this context is not new, and has been used to describe abdominal contamination, infection and sepsis (Schein *et al*, 1997).

Quantification of bioburden may prove difficult, as clinical outcomes rely on the ability of the host to mount an immune response, and this will be different for each individual. Progression along the continuum in the direction of increasing clinical severity denotes increasing bioburden, which only becomes clinically relevant for chronicity once the state of colonisation has been passed. It is crucial to remember that in the wound healing by secondary intention, colonisation is the 'healthy' situation (Edwards and Harding, 2004). Colonised wounds heal, often without the need to control bioburden artificially by means of antimicrobial manoeuvres, because the host immune response is adequate on its own (Leaper, 1994).

The most controversial point on the continuum is that of critical colonisation; a state of delayed healing. This has now been rationalised in a scientific study by Stephens *et al* (2003). Although the authors did not claim this to be the case, their findings strongly suggest that soluble metabolites from anaerobic cocci can give rise to 'delayed healing', through the impaired metabolism of key wound cell populations. Clinical management has been defined as a need for topical, sustained release antimicrobial (not antibiotic) wound dressings (Kingsley, 2003; Bolton and Hermans, 2004).

The quantity and diversity of microbes representing the states of colonisation, critical colonisation, and infection, are individual and dependent on the quality of the host immune response. Some wounds progress quickly from colonisation to infection via a clinically indistinct 'critical colonisation' state. Other wounds stop at that point and become indolent (Heggers *et al*, 1992; Ennis and Meneses, 2000). Critically colonised wounds will become increasingly 'chronic', or indolent, because cellular cascades are disordered and there is a biochemical imbalance arising from bacterial metabolism (Wall *et al*, 2002; Stephens *et al*, 2003). Once that is established, wounds in this state can prove resistant to adjustment with current therapy, as well as emerging novel therapies such as protease inhibitors, extracellular matrix components, and topical growth factors. Thus, early recognition of disordered healing caused commonly, either wholly or partly, by microbes, is vital to achieving good outcomes.

Infection, critical colonisation and colonisation

The Wound Infection Continuum has historically been drawn to show increasing severity of clinical and microbiological states, from left to right (Kingsley, 2001). It can be reversed to link with the Wound Healing and Exudate Continuums, so providing a 'global' wound assessment of key presenting features: healing (tissues in the wound); infection (wound bioburden); and, exudate (Gray *et al*, 2005) to promote ease of assessment and documentation of progress in clinical practice. In the original Infection Continuum (Kingsley, 2001), the states of 'sterility' and 'contamination' were included to reflect the presence of microbial growth from the outset of wounding. Sterility represents the absence of any organism in the wound and is a very unusual situation in wounds healing by secondary intent (Leaper, 1994). For the purpose of clinical practice, this state can be ignored. Similarly, contamination, which means presence of organisms with no active growth and not accompanied by a visible host response, is of no relevance to clinical practice.

The normal microbiological state of a healing wound is that of colonisation, representing a stable state where growth and death of organisms is balanced or below the immune system's healing disruption threshold (Isenberg, 1998; Heinzelmann *et al*, 2002).

Some authors differentiate infection into 'local' and 'systemic' (Sibbald *et al*, 2000; Edwards and Harding, 2004). This classification has been used to provide guidance on the route of administration for systemic antibiotics. Schultz *et al* (2003) describe four levels of microbial interaction:

- contamination
- colonisation
- critical colonisation
- infection.

Edwards and Harding (2004) include two further levels:

- spreading invasive infection
- septicaemia.

Dow *et al* (1999) and Schultz *et al* (2003) define, with other factors, a ring of cellulitis of <2cm to suggest antibiotic treatment via oral route, with extensive cellulitis (by absence of further definition presumed to be >2cm) requiring intravenous therapy.

The choice of route of antibiotic delivery is linked to the time taken to achieve a therapeutic level of antibiotics at the site, with intravenous delivery naturally being faster than oral administration. Intravenous therapy is indicated in the more severe cases where the consequences of systemic infection can be grave, eg. lymphoedema (Keeley, 2000). It seems logical to relate the extent of the inflammation with the severity of infection and provide guidance for intervention, but to our knowledge, the choice of the 2cm threshold and therapeutic response are not yet validated by published research.

The use of the word 'systemic' for infection that has spread beyond 2cm from the wound edge could also be unintentionally misleading. Some wounds have wider zones of peripheral redness but remain local in character, meaning that the inflammation zone does not continue to extend and the patient does not exhibit systemic infection signs produced by the consequences of bacteraemia, notably fever, rigor, and positive blood culture. Therefore, for the purposes of reconsidering the states to depict on the Wound Infection Continuum, the terms 'local' and 'spreading' infection will be used, denoted by the 2cm threshold as previously discussed in the literature. Further information on this can be found in *Table 3.1*.

The remaining state lies between colonisation and infection and is called critical colonisation (Davis, 1998; Schultz *et al*, 2003; Edwards and Harding, 2004). This state has also been referred to as covert infection (Dow *et al*, 1999; Dow, 2001), or localised infection (Gardner *et al*, 2001). Indeed, the so-called 'stunned' wound (ie. a wound that begins on a normal healing trajectory and then plateaus, becoming recalcitrant) could be critically colonised (Ennis and Meneses, 2000). However, some authorities claim that critical colonisation could equally be described as 'sub-clinical' infection (George *et al*, 2001). These terms are used to identify different states of microbiological and immunological activity. The change from one state to another depends on many factors (*Table 3.2*).

Each successive stage from left to right on the Continuum (*Figure 3.9*) involves an increase in the quantity of microbes, a new pathogen arrival, an increase in the quantity of virulent organisms, or an increase in the virulence (Wilson *et al*, 2002) of the collective species mixture through bacterial synergy (Bowler *et al*, 2001). The situation may shift in favour of the microorganisms if the host immune response is impaired or suddenly reduced (Bowler, 2002; Heinzelmann *et al*, 2002). In addition, shift may result from the presence of potentiating factors such as the introduction of foreign bodies that reduce the necessary inoculum needed to produce a worsening microbiological environment.

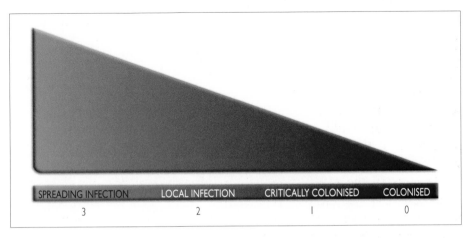

SPREADING INFECTION	LOCAL INFECTION	CRITICALLY COLONISED	COLONISED
3	2	I	0

Figure 3.9: The Wound Infection Continuum

Identifying and obtaining treatment objectives

The Wound Infection Continuum is a useful adjunct to the identification of treatment objectives (Gray *et al*, 2005). At different stages of the Continuum there is likely to be the need for a different treatment objective. It is, however, vital that the identification of such objectives is only arrived at once a full assessment of the patient has taken place and the implications of the presence of systemic illness or disability understood.

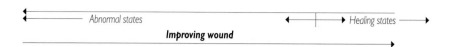

Table 3.1: Revised Wound Infection Continuum with diagnostic and treatment information				
	Spreading infection	Local infection	Critical colonisation	Colonisation
Key local characteristics	>2cm redness with pain (unless insensate).	2cm or less redness with pain. Sudden necrosis on wound bed (red inflammatory zone may not be present).	Static (despite appropriate therapy). No cellulitis.	Expected progression towards healing. No cellulitis (but may be small degree of inflammation in early stages consistent with inflammatory phase – generally not more painful to pressure than background wound pain)
Other local characteristics	Heat. Swelling.	Heat and swelling (can be difficult to identify in small red inflammatory zone).		
Additional local characteristics that may be present in addition to key ones	Extension to main wound at skin level. Blistering (fluid filled). New satellite wounds in red inflammatory zone. Increased wetness. Haemorrhagic patching or spotting in surrounding skin. Purulent exudate*. Maceration, if control of exudate is inadequate. Extensive necrotic and/or sloughing necrotic tissue.	Extension to main wound at skin level. Extension to wound at its base (pocketing). Increased wetness. Purulent exudate*. Maceration if control of exudates is inadequate. Extensive necrotic and/or sloughing necrotic tissue. Discolouration of granulation tissue (darkening). Friable bleeding granulation tissue (possibly with very bright red tissue). Foul odour.	Thick slough not responding to standard debridement techniques. Fast returning thick slough after sharp or maggot debridement. Wet wound. Purulent exudates. Maceration if control of exudate is inadequate. Blue/green exudate (Pseudomonas aeruginosa). Foul odour. Discolouration of granulation tissue (darkening). Friable bleeding granulation tissue (possibly with very bright red tissue).	Debride damaged tissue under standard therapeutic approaches. Gently moist wound surface. Slough but light and mobile in consistency. Inflammation from initial wounding consistent with expectation for inflammation phase of wound healing, but fading away or gone if wound older. Granulation tissue of healthy red colour. Epithelial tissue with colour different from, but relevant to, normal skin tone. Reducing wound size in last 1–2 weeks.

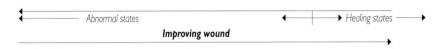

Abnormal states ← → Healing states →

Improving wound →

Table 3.1: continued

	Spreading infection	Local infection	Critical colonisation	Colonisation
Possible systemic features	Neutrophilia. Rising C-reactive protein. Fever. Rigors. Confusion (in the elderly). Bacteraemia. Tachycardia. Tachypnoea. Lymphangiitis. Lymphadenitis.	Neutrophilia. Rising C-reactive protein.	None.	None.
Suggested treatment	Systemic antibiotics – oral if red zone static and still localised even if >2cm – IV if red zone more than an obvious local ring around wound or if actively spreading. Use local formulary. Consider topical antiseptic dressings – at this stage medicated dressings may not be cost- or clinically-effective, though it is clinically reasonable to use them in the diabetic foot ulcer, critically ischaemic wounds, burns, and the severely immuno-compromised patient.	Systemic antibiotics – oral. Use local formulary. Topical antiseptic dressings – normally iodine or silver in formulation, or combination suitable for wet wounds. Locally infected wounds with a necrotic eschar will need a wetter formulation. Adjunctive measures – rapid debridement of necrotic tissue may be necessary, consider relevant strategy, eg. sharp or surgical.	Topical antiseptic dressings – normally iodine or silver in formulation or combination suitable for wet wound. Slow-release formulations are preferred. Medical grade Manuka honey may be considered, especially to control foul odour. Use local formulary. Consider topical antiseptic irrigations – some authors suggest use of dilute vinegar to control *Pseudomonas* if blue/green exudate is present. Adjunctive measures – debridement of necrotic tissue may be necessary. Consider relevant strategy, eg. maggots. Use of anti-protease therapy may be valuable with antimicrobials.	Standard wound therapy and control of underlying aetiological factors (eg. venous hypertension, forces of pressure) as local guidelines. Topical antiseptic dressings – normally, no antimicrobials are necessary, however, prophylaxis may be considered in vulnerable wound groups, such as diabetic foot ulcers or vulnerable immuno-suppressed patients. It can also be considered if the patient has a recurrent history of infection in this wound.

* 'Wound exudate need not be purulent in the setting of infection, as bacterial phospholipases and other enzymes and toxins can rapidly destroy neutrophils, producing the classical watery exudate or "dishwater" pus seen in polymicrobial necrotizing infections'. Dow *et al,* 1999

Table 3.2: Wound treatments and their use across the Wound Infection Continuum

Mode of action	Product	Spreading infection	Local infection	Critically colonised	Colonised
Active	Alginates with silver				
	Film with silver				
	Cadexomer iodine				
	Hydrocolloids with silver				
	Honey				
	Hydrogel sheets with honey				
	Hydrofiber® with silver				
	Iodine tulle				
	Nanocrystaline silver cloth				
	Silver sulphadiazine cream				
Passive	Activated charcoal cloth				
	Foam with silver				

Spreading infection: remove blood stream infection and reduce wound and surrounding tissue bioburden

A spreading infection should be recognised as a serious systemic illness, and appropriate medical management sought at the earliest point. As such, the choice of dressing will have little impact on the spreading infection. A systemic response in the form of antibiotics is likely to be the treatment of choice and the wound dressing can seek only to reduce the level of bacteria at the wound surface and thus help prevent re-infection.

Localised infection: remove infection from surrounding tissue and reduce wound bioburden

Where the wound is identified as locally infected, there are a number of options open to the practitioner. Some authors suggest that a localised infection can be treated using topical antimicrobials alone without recourse to antibiotics (European Pressure Ulcer Advisory Panel [EPUAP], 1999). Others, however, recommend the use of topical antimicrobials with oral antibiotics (Kingsley, 2005). Where the practitioner is satisfied that the patient's overall condition does not suggest a high risk of the infection developing into a spreading infection, it would seem reasonable to adopt a topical antimicrobial-only approach. However, the practitioner should remain alert to the possibility of an advancement of the infection and be prepared to alter the treatment as required. Also, it would be valuable to set a period of time from the outset in which a reduction of signs and symptoms of infection would be expected to start (eg. <7 days or perhaps by the return of swab culture results), as it would not be appropriate to unnecessarily allow continuation of pain, or the potential for wound bed deterioration.

Critical colonisation: reduce wound bioburden

Critically colonised wounds require a reduction in the level of bacteria in the wound to allow progression to healing. The topical application of an antimicrobial is probably the most effective way in which to reduce the critically colonised wound bioburden to levels that allow the wound to heal (Cooper, 2004).

Colonised: maintain wound bioburden

Wounds that are identified as colonised do not require any form of topical antimicrobial as the wound bioburden is in a healthy state. Only where there are concerns regarding the patient's immune response, or overall medical condition, should topical antimicrobials be used prophylactically; for example, wounds with a history of recurrent infection, including some diabetic foot ulceration and wounds on lymphoedematous limbs. The indiscriminate prophylactic use of antimicrobials is to be discouraged.

Wound products used to obtain treatment objectives

Topical antimicrobial dressings are varied in their form of presentation and action in the wound. As a result there exists a large range of products suitable to aid the practitioner in the achievement of Wound Infection Continuum treatment objectives. In the interest of clarity, the authors have sought to categorise the wound treatments available into two distinct groups: active and passive. These terms describe the mode of the respective dressings, as some dressings donate antimicrobial properties into the wound (active) and others seek to act upon the bacteria as they pass into the dressing (passive). Each form of dressing has its place and it is for practitioners to decide upon the action they require, and the product they select, based on a holistic assessment of the patient.

While the wound dressings available can be divided into two distinct groups by mode of action, there still remain differences in the form such dressings take. In *Table 3.2* the authors present the dressings in terms of the mode of action, type (eg. Hydrofiber®) and where they may be used across the Wound Infection Continuum. As with any dressing selection, the practitioner must be satisfied that the selection process includes a full assessment of the patient and a full understanding of the actions of the dressing.

Accurate assessment of a wound's bioburden, and the impact of bacteria on the wound, are essential components of wound management. The Wound Infection Continuum encourages practitioners to categorise the level of wound bioburden and identify the relevant treatment objectives. Once treatment objectives have been identified, it is important that the practitioner is comfortable that any treatments selected are appropriate for the patient. It is also important to recognise that topical treatments can only be effective when used appropriately, and that their potential to impact on the wound is not misunderstood.

Topical antimicrobials will not eradicate a spreading infection, and such cases require urgent medical intervention. However, topical antimicrobials are of benefit in the reduction of wound bioburden, and have a leading role to play in the eradication of local infections and in cases of critical colonisation (Bolton and Hermans, 2004; Bowler *et al*, 2001). Where the decision is taken to treat a local infection without recourse to antibiotics, the practitioner should be confident that the patient has been appropriately assessed. This can only be achieved following a full assessment of the patient as a whole, taking into consideration his/her physical, psychological and social circumstances.

Conclusion

The Wound Infection Continuum offers the practitioner the means to approach assessment of the wound's bioburden in a systematic manner. This leads to the identification of clear treatment objectives. The practitioner is faced with a wide variety of products that can be of benefit in the achievement of treatment objectives, and it is important that such choices are made in the full knowledge of the patient's requirements and the product's abilities.

Part IV: Using The Wound Exudate Continuum to aid wound assessment

Wound healing occurs in four overlapping phases: haemostasis; inflammation; granulation/epithelialisation; and tissue remodelling (Davidson, 1992). Upon injury, vasoconstriction occurs with the aim of reducing blood loss. Haemostasis is achieved by the formation of a clot, which seals the wound. Following haemostasis, the inflammatory process begins, during which wound exudate is produced by the tissues surrounding the wound. Normal serous exudate is essential to the healing of the wound (Field and Kerstein, 1994). However, wound exudate is not always 'normal' in terms of volume and/or consistency; it can present significant management challenges and be a sign of underlying problems relating to the wound bioburden (Cutting and Harding, 1994; Gilchrist, 1999; Vowden and Vowden, 2003, 2004; Cutting, 2004).

Where a wound is healing without complication, exudate can be considered a normal feature. It is produced when blood vessels dilate, post-haemostasis, as part of the inflammatory process. Endothelial cells swell, and so open gaps in the vessel wall permitting extravasation of serous fluid. The presence of this fluid in the tissues surrounding the wound contributes to localised pain, heat, and swelling; symptoms that are associated with inflammation.

Normal wound exudate is mainly composed of three elements: serous fluid from the leaking blood vessels; debris from local damaged tissue; and growth factors or cytokines (Chen *et al*, 1992; Rogers *et al*, 1995; Cutting, 2004). Wound exudate has a key role to play in the moist wound-healing process as it provides not only moisture, but also components which support the removal of dead tissue and the formation of new tissue. Factors such as the underlying condition of the patient, dressing selection, and the pathology of the wound, all affect the production of exudate (White, 2001). Wound exudate has been shown to contain different components at different stages of healing, ie. acute wounds contain growth factors and chronic wounds contain tissue-degrading enzymes (White, 2001; Cutting, 2004).

Exudate can present significant management challenges. For example, in the case of venous leg ulcers and pressure ulcers, protease enzymes contained in chronic wound exudate (Chen *et al*, 1992) can, if they come into contact with the surrounding skin, result in the development of excoriation and maceration (Cameron and Powell, 1992). Large quantities of exudate can saturate the wound bed (Lamke *et al*, 1997) and peri-wound area, causing further maceration (Cutting, 1999; White and Cutting, 2003). Wound exudate can also increase the risk of infection if it soaks through a dressing, thus allowing bacteria to 'strike-through' the wound dressing (this is the passage of exudate from the wound bed through a permeable dressing to appear at the dressing surface – it is believed to be an avenue for bacterial contamination from the environment) . However, wound exudate can promote healing if it is managed to maintain an optimum moist environment, and avoid damage to surrounding skin (Bishop *et al*, 2003).

Exudate will be found at some point in all wounds healing by secondary intention. The volume and viscosity of wound exudate produced by the wound will be influenced by the stage of healing, and the presence or absence of factors such as infection. Wounds healing by secondary intention and without complication will gradually reduce their production of exudate as the healing process progresses.

Assessing exudate

Traditionally, exudate has been described in terms of its perceived volume, eg. as light/low, moderate, or heavy (Watret, 1997). This form of assessment is very subjective and difficult to quantify in the absence of significant investigation, such as the weighing of dressings pre- and post-use (Thomas, 1997). Vowden and Vowden (2003, 2004) suggest that exudate volume should not be viewed in isolation, but in conjunction with viscosity. By considering both these aspects, an insight can be gained into the underlying condition of the wound and of the patient. They are indicative of the infection status (Cutting, 2004).

The authors suggest that wound exudate volume and viscosity be assessed by:

- considering the exudate that is retained within the dressing
- noting the number of dressing changes required in forty-eight hours
- visual inspection of the wound.

This approach to assessment is complementary to current management strategies, such as the six 'Cs' as proposed by Vowden and Vowden (2003) (*Table 3.3*).

Table 3.3: Exudate management strategy based on six 'Cs', adapted from Vowden and Vowden, 2004					
Cause	Control	Components	Containment	Correction	Complications
Systemic	Whether effective systemic or local control possible	Bacterial	Dressing seal. At the wound surface, with the dressing and away from the wound	Bioburden control	Skin protection
		Necrotic			Protein loss
		Chemical composition		Debride-ment	Pain
Local					Odour
Wound-related		Volume and viscosity			
		pH			

The Wound Exudate Continuum (*Figure 3.10*) is offered as an aid to quantifying the volume and viscosity of wound exudate. The gradings for both of these features are 'high', 'medium' and 'low', and allow wound exudate to be categorised by a numerical score. For example, a wound with exudate of low volume and of medium viscosity would be in the low/medium category and would score 4 (placing it in the low exudate [green] portion of the Continuum). Any score in the green zone should be seen as advantageous to wound healing.

If the wound exudate score is 6, this places the wound in the amber zone. Wounds that are assessed as being in the amber zone require careful consideration as this category could either indicate an improvement or deterioration in the wound's condition. For example, if the previous recording had been in the green zone, then the practitioner should seek to identify why the wound has moved (deteriorated) into the amber zone. A change in score to red from amber, ie. a deterioration, may be because of an alteration in the wound bioburden, indicating critical colonisation or the development of an infection. However, if the previous score had been in the red zone, an amber score would indicate an improvement in the condition of the wound. Any score in the red zone should be investigated urgently as this may indicate local or spreading infection, particularly if the previous score had not been in this zone.

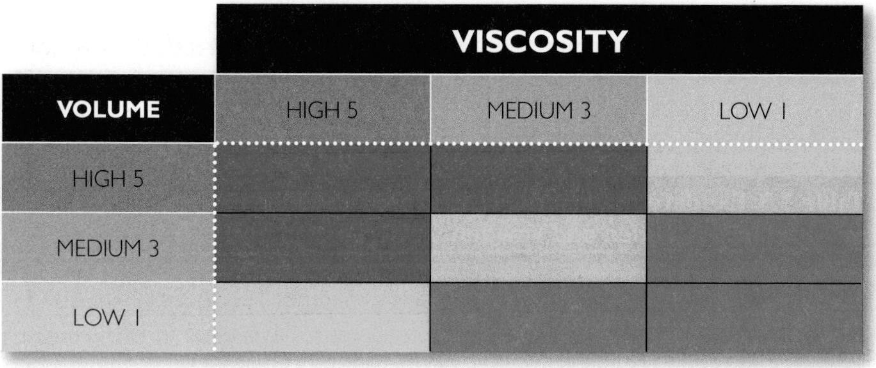

VOLUME	VISCOSITY		
	HIGH 5	MEDIUM 3	LOW 1
HIGH 5			
MEDIUM 3			
LOW 1			

Figure 3.10: The Wound Exudate Continuum

Identifying and obtaining treatment objectives

When reviewing the wound, the exudate on the dressing and present in the wound should be assessed using the questions outlined in *Table 3.4*. This is a highly subjective assessment and should be used to guide clinical judgement, not replace it. Any wound assessed as having both high viscosity and high volume of wound exudate would score a full ten points and be regarded as causing serious concern. The overriding aim of the Wound Exudate Continuum is to encourage a systematic approach to wound care and to support clinical decision-making. Regardless of the zone, the assessment points to the treatment objectives will fall into one of three categories:

1. Absorbing moisture
2. Maintaining current moisture balance
3. Donating moisture.

When these objectives are added to the objectives identified using the Wound Healing and Wound Infection Continuums, a clear picture of the overall treatment objectives is achieved.

Table 3.4: Exudate assessment: questions to ask	
Questions	Answers
How often has the dressing been changed over the past 48 hours?	Provides an indication as to the volume of exudate being produced
Has there been any leakage from the dressing?	This may provide information on the suitability of the dressing used, and give an indication of the volumes of exudate being produced
Is there any residue on the surface of the wound dressing?	High viscosity exudate is likely to be found on the surface of a wound dressing
Have the margins become macerated?	Maceration is usually associated with high volumes of exudate, and/or prolonged wear time
Is there any exudate on the wound bed?	High viscosity exudate is more likely to be found adhering to the wound bed
Can the staff or patient offer any information regarding the nature of exudate observed over 48 hours?	Often an asssessment is difficult because dressings have been removed or the patient bathed before an assessment

Once an assessment has been carried out using the Wound Exudate Continuum and a colour zone identified, it is possible to identify which product may be suitable using *Figure 3.11*. In *Figure 3.11* the products have been divided according to their primary function, and placed in the zones of the continuum in which they have been identified to function by their manufacturers. Those products with an antimicrobial function have been identified with an asterisk. This may be particularly useful where an infection or critical colonisation is thought to be present.

Function	Product	Red	Amber	Green
Devices/dressings				
	Topical negative pressure	■	■	■
	Wound Manager™	■		
Primary dressings				
	Alginates *	■	■	■
	Capillary	■	■	■
	Hydrofiber®*	■	■	■
Primary/secondary dressings				
	Foams*	■	■	
	Films*			■
	Hydrocolloids* #			■
	Hydrofiber®*	■	■	■
	Hydrogels* #		■	■

Figure 3.11: Exudate management options
* Denotes where some of the products within this category contain an antimicrobial function
# Denotes products which can donate moisture to the wound where there is insufficient moisture

Product functions

Device/dressings

In *Figure 3.11*, the first category of products are those which can be described as device/dressings. In this category there are two different products. First, topical negative pressure, which works by applying negative pressure to a wound bed and thus removing the exudate via a tube to a canister. This product can function across the spectrum of exudate zones. A Wound Manager™ (ConvaTec) is a device which is similar in construction to a colostomy bag, and acts as a reservoir where there are large amounts of exudate. This product is limited to the red zone, and, in some cases, the amber zone. Generally, the wound manager has a short-term application in acute situations such as dehisced abdominal wounds.

Primary dressings

In this category, the dressings are applied directly to the wound bed and absorb exudate. Two of the dressings in this section have an antimicrobial function; namely, the alginates and Hydrofiber®. The other dressing, the capillary dressing, has no antimicrobial function but has a large capacity to absorb and wick fluid away from the wound bed. All of the dressings in this category require a secondary dressing to cover them.

Primary/secondary dressings

The dressings in this category can be applied either as a primary dressing which does not require a secondary dressing, such as the hydrocolloids, hydrogel sheets or film dressings. The foam dressings can act as a primary dressing but are also frequently used as secondary dressings absorbing exudate which has passed through the primary dressing. Once again, some products found within these categories contain an antimicrobial function and some do not. In this category there are products which can also donate moisture to the wound bed if required.

Conclusion

The Wound Exudate Continuum provides the user with a systematic approach to wound exudate, going beyond simply guessing the volume of exudate produced. The Wound Exudate Continuum promotes the view that exudate can shed light on the health of the wound and assists in the identification of different levels of wound bioburden. It can also facilitate the identification of clear treatment objectives which, when used with the other aspects of the Applied Wound Management system, can deliver a full wound assessment.

Considering wound exudate in terms of its viscosity and volume, a valuable insight into the wound's underlying condition can be obtained. The Wound Exudate Continuum is designed to provide the practitioner with a method of assessment based on estimation of viscosity and volume of exudate, which relates to the underlying condition of the wound. Its use is intended as part of a thorough assessment and should be used within the Applied Wound Management (Gray *et al*, 2005) framework. The values attached to the different levels of exudate are designed to provide the practitioner with an aid to assessment, and not to replace sound clinical decision-making.

Part V: Using AWM in the clinical setting

Following the application of the three continuums, the wound can be defined in terms of:

- tissue/colour (WHC)
- bioburden/host response (WIC)
- exudate volume/consistency (WEC).

It is at this stage that consideration must be given to the cause (aetiology) of the wound. Such an assessment would, for example, in the case of a heel pressure ulcer, necessitate a very different form of management/treatment than if it were a leg ulcer or a diabetic foot ulcer. Each wound would require treatment/management relevant to the underlying pathology, despite recording the same initial results following AWM assessment by the three continuums. To summarise, when using AWM, assess:

- healing (WHC)
- bioburden (WIC)
- exudate (WEC)
- wound type/aetiology
- underlying pathology.

Table 3.5 gives further examples of this type of decision-making and the two cases studies that follow illustrate the use of the AWM framework.

Table 3.5: Using Applied Wound Management

Wound Continuum	Treatment objectives	Patient assessment	Wound type	Treatment
Healing = black Infection = colonised Exudate = low/low *(Figure 3.13, p. 91)*	Debride Maintain Hydrate	A frail individual with a poor overall condition due to CVA*. Poor prognosis	Pressure ulcer to heel	Hydrocolloid change every 5–7 days, or sheet hydrogel change every 2–3 days, or amorphous hydrogel change every 2 days.
			Prevent further damage by using a heel protector device	Heel protector *in situ* at all times
Healing = yellow/red Infection = locally infected Exudate = low/medium *(Figure 3.15, p. 93)*	Debride/ promote granulation Reduce bacterial load	As above	Debride tissue while promoting	Alginate/ Hydrofiber® with anti-microbial properties or cadexomer, iodine or honey ointment
			Manage local infection/prevent spreading infection	Absorb exudate Absorbent foam dressing to cover

* CVA = cerebral vascular accident

Conclusion

Applied Wound Management seeks to utilise three continuums to facilitate wound assessment (Gray *et al*, 2005). When this system is used in conjunction with an accurate diagnosis of the pathology of the wound, the practitioner is in an informed position to identify treatment objectives and monitor the effects of the treatment by measuring the clinical outcomes against the original assessment. Four tools have been developed to facilitate this process. An overview of each and how best to utilise these tools to facilitate wound healing/management is given in the *Appendix (pp. 113–119)*.

Case study I

An eighty-five-year-old male was admitted to orthopoedics with a fractured neck of femur. On assessment he also presented with a partial-thickness dermal burn to his left shoulder blade area. The wound measured 12cm x 5cm on initial assessment.

WHC

Figure 3.12 illustrates the wound presenting with a deep dermal burn of black/yellow tissue, which needs rehydrating to facilitate the debridement of the devitalised tissue.

Figure 3.13 illustrates an improvement in the wound bed condition, with debridement of necrotic tissue. However, reference to the Wound Healing Continuum still demonstrates that there is black/yellow/red and pink tissue present. Of primary importance is the black tissue, followed secondly by the yellow. The treatment aim is to focus on the debridement of the black/yellow tissue by rehydration.

WIC

The Wound Infection Continuum offers the reader the opportunity to consider if the wound has altered healing due to the presence of bacteria. In both images there are no signs of local or spreading infection. The wound is progressing and improving which would rule out any form of critical colonisation. However, the wound is a chronic wound which was caused by a burn, therefore, the wound will be colonised, but this will not inhibit healing.

WEC

Review of *Figures 3.12* and *3.13* show that there are low volumes of exudate with low viscosity. This indicates that exudate management is not a problem with this wound and can be categorised as 'low'. However, to facilitate debridement, a degree of moisture should be provided by the dressing. Once black/yellow tissue begins to soften, there may be an increase in the levels of exudate, but this does not indicate an infection according to the Wound Infection Continuum.

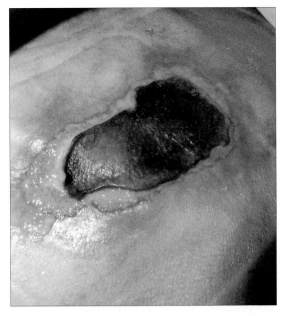

Figure 3.12: Burn at presentation

Summary

In summary, the wound presents as 'black/yellow', therefore requiring debridement. The wound is 'colonised', with 'low' exudate levels and 'low' viscosity. The wound should be managed by application of a dressing which facilities

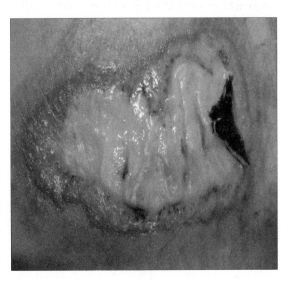

Figure 3.13: Burn at first review

debridement by providing a moist environment (ie. autolytic), but which is not required to absorb exudate or to have any antimicrobial properties.

Case study 2

A seventy-five-year-old female who was cared for in a long-term care of the elderly unit following a cerebral vascular event, presented with a pressure ulcer to her right heel. This occurred due to a deterioration in her physical condition, despite deploying all preventative strategies.

WHC

According to the WHC, the wound shown in *Figure 3.14* is clearly 100% black necrotic tissue. Therefore, the initial management of this wound is to facilitate debridement of this devitalised tissue. *Figure 3.15* shows that debridement of the black tissue has occurred and that the wound now presents as a yellow/red wound. The colour of importance now is yellow, with debridement of the yellow tissue pivotal to the wound's ongoing progress. The presence of red tissue indicates that the wound is reaching a stage where debridement can stop and stimulation of granulation can occur.

WIC

The initial picture (*Figure 3.14*) is of a moist, black wound. There are no clinical signs of infection, but the wound is malodorous. The odour is due to the presence of anaerobes, but does not indicate that the wound is infected. In fact, the wound is colonised because, as yet, no healing delay has occurred. *Figure 3.15* shows a wound that is critically colonised — categorised as such, since it has stayed in this 'dormant' condition for a number of weeks without any sign of improvement. The treatment required is the application of a topical antimicrobial to reduce the bioburden and to 'kick-start' the healing process. No systemic antibiotics are necessary.

WEC

The wound started off with low levels of low viscosity exudate, scoring as 'low' on the continuum, but, as the wound progressed, the levels and the viscosity increased to warrant a 'medium' score. This change in exudate should act as a prompt to the clinician that a change has occurred, and a review of current treatment should be triggered. The wound is 'critically colonised' (*Figure 3.15*) according to the WIC and, therefore, treatment with an antimicrobial should be commenced. As there is an increased level of exudate, an appropriate absorbent secondary dressing should be considered.

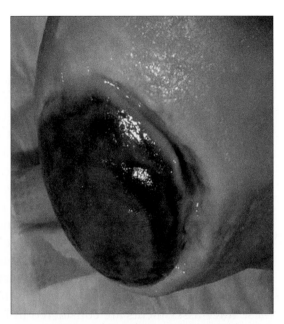

Figure 3.14: Heel ulcer at presentation

Summary

In summary, the wound started off as a 'black wound' with no infection and minimal exudate. As debridement proceeded, the wound changed to a 'yellow/red wound' that was critically colonised due to non-healing and the presence of bacteria, which led to an increase in the levels of exudate.

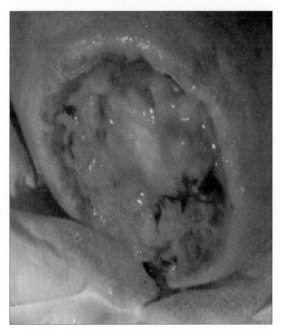

Figure 3.15: Heel ulcer at first review

Conclusion

At the centre of the AWM framework is the WHC, which has attempted to address the shortcomings of previous colour-based assessment tools. It recognises the variance in colour and requires the practitioner to rate the wound according to the colour closest to the left of the continuum. The WIC is aimed at providing a structure and logic to wound bioburden assessment as, with the WHC, the aim is to move the wound status to the right of the continuum. The WEC addresses exudate as an indicator of the wound condition, and needs the user to rate both the viscosity and volume of the exudate. Once this assessment has been completed, the exudate rating will fall into one of three categories, giving an indication as to the wound's underlying condition. When all three Continuum ratings are taken together, they provide the practitioner with a clear, logical and coherent assessment of the condition of the wound. Only when these three assessments are considered in light of the type of wound, its underlying pathology, and the key principles of its management, can the practitioner design an appropriate treatment/management plan.

The principles of WBP and TIME are now recognised as new paradigms in wound management, and it is up to those active in the field to interpret these concepts in a manner relevant to their own clinical practice. The AWM framework is the authors' response to the need to develop a more systematic and practical approach to wound assessment.

The AWM system can be of benefit to those less familiar with wound healing/management by introducing a systematic approach to decision-making. For the specialist practitioner, utilising the framework facilitates clinical audit, and the supporting software can generate relevant clinical data. Whatever the level of knowledge of the practitioner, the AWM system can facilitate systematic clinical decision-making and clinical audit of practice.

References

Argenta LC, Morykwas MJ (1997) Vacuum-assisted closure: a new method for treatment: Clinical Experience. *Annals Plastic Surg* **38**(6): 563–76

Bale S (1997) A guide to wound debridement. *J Wound Care* **6**: 179–82

Banwell PE (1999) Topical negative pressure therapy in wound care. *J Wound Care* **8**(2): 79–84

Bishop SM, Walker M, Rogers AA, Chen WYJ (2003) Importance of moisture balance at the wound–dressing interface. *J Wound Care* **12**(4): 125–8

Bolton L, Hermans MHE (2004) How do we manage critically colonized wounds? *Rehabil Nurs* **29**(6): 187–94

Bowler PG (2002) Wound pathophysiology, infection and therapeutic options. *Ann Med* **34**(6): 419–27

Bowler P, Duerden B, Armstrong D (2001) Wound microbiology and associated approaches to wound management. *Clin Microbiol Rev* **14**(2): 244–69

Browne A, Dow G, Sibbald RG (2001) Infected wounds: definitions and controversies. In: Falanga V, ed. *Cutaneous Wound Healing*. Martin Dunitz, London

Cameron J, Powell S (1992) Contact dermatitis: its importance in leg ulcer patients. *Wound Management* **2**(3): 12–13

Chen WY, Rogers AA, Lydon MJ (1992) Characterization of biologic properties of wound fluid collected during early stages of wound healing. *J Invest Dermatol* **99**(5): 559–64

Colebrook L, Lowbury EJ, Hurst L (1960) The growth and death of wound bacteria in serum, exudate and slough. *J Hyg (Lond)* **58**: 357–66

Cooper RA (2004) http://www.worldwidewounds.com/2004/february/Cooper/Topical-Antimicrobial-Agents.html

Cooper P, Russell F, Stringfellow S (2003) Modern wound management: an update of common products. *Nurs Residential Care* **5**(7): 322–34

Cutting KF (1999) The causes and prevention of maceration of the skin. *J Wound Care* **8**(4): 200–2

Cutting KF (2003) Wound healing, bacteria and topical therapies. *EWMA Journal* **3**(1): 17–19

Cutting KF (2004) Wound exudate. In: White RJ, ed. *Trends in Wound Care, vol III*. Quay Books, MA Healthcare Ltd, London

Cutting K, Harding KG (1994) Criteria for identifying wound infection. *J Wound Care* **3**(4): 198–201

Cutting KF, White RJ (2005) Criteria for identifying wound infection: revisited. *Ostomy Wound Management* **5**(1): 28–34

Cuzzell JZ (1988) The new red, yellow, black color code. *Am J Nurs* **88**(10): 1342–46

Davidson JM (1992) Wound repair. In: Gallin JI, Goldstein IM, Snyderman R, eds. *Inflammation: Basic Principles and Clinical Correlates*. 2nd edn. Raven Press, New York: 809–19

Davies P (2004) Current thinking on the management of necrotic and sloughy wounds. *Prof Nurse* **19**(10): 34–6

Davis E (1998) Education, microbiology and chronic wounds. *J Wound Care* **7**(6): 272–4

Dealey C (1994) *The Care of Wounds. A Guide for Nurses*. Blackwell Science, Oxford

de Peyrolle M (2002) Colour evaluation of wounds. *Rev Infirm* **80**: 31–2

Dow G (2001) Infection in chronic wounds. In: Krasner D, Rodeheaver G, Sibbald RG, eds. *Chronic Wound Care: A Clinical Source Book for Healthcare Professionals*. 3rd edn. HMP Communications, Wayne, PA

Dow G, Browne A, Sibbald RG (1999) Infection in chronic wounds: controversies in diagnosis and treatment. *Ostomy Wound Management* **45**(8): 23–7, 29–40

Dowsett C, Ayello E (2004) TIME principles of chronic wound bed preparation and treatment. *Br J Nurs* **13**(15): S16–23

Dowsett C, Edwards-Jones V, Davies S (2004) Infection control for wound bed preparation. *Br J Community Nurs Supplement* **9**(9): TIME Suppl 12–17

Edwards R, Harding KG (2004) Bacteria and wound healing. *Curr Opin Infect Dis* **17**(2): 91–6

Ennis W, Meneses P (2000) Wound healing at the local level: the stunned wound. *Ostomy Wound Management* **46**(1A Suppl): 39S–48S

European Pressure Ulcer Advisory Panel (1999) Guidelines on treatment of pressure ulcers. *EPUAP Review* **1**(2): 31–3

European Tissue Repair Society (2003) Statements on important aspects of wound healing. *ETRS Bulletin* **10**: 2–3

European Wound Management Association (2005) *Identifying criteria for wound infection*. Position Document. EWMA, London

Fletcher J (2003) The benefits of applying wound bed preparation into practice. *J Wound Care* **12**(9): 347–9

Field C, Kerstein M (1994) Overview of wound healing in a moist environment. *Am J Surg* **167**(Suppl 1a): S25–S30

Finlay BB, Falkow S (1997) Common themes in microbial pathogenicity revisited. *Microbiol Mol Biol Rev* **61**(2): 136–69

Gardner SE, Frantz RA, Doebbeling BN (2001) The validity of the clinical signs and symptoms used to identify localized chronic wound infection. *Wound Rep Regen* **9**(3): 178–86

George A, Bang RL, Lari AR (2001) Acute thrombocytopenic crisis following burns complicated by staphylococcal septicaemia. *Burns* **27**(1): 84–8

Gilchrist B (1999) Wound infection. In: Miller M, Glover D, eds. *Wound Management: Theory and Practice*. NT Books, London

Goldman RJ, Salcido R (2002) More than one way to measure a wound: an overview of tools and techniques. *Adv Skin Wound Care* **15**(5): 236–43

Gray D, White RJ, Cooper P (2003) The wound healing continuum. In: White RJ, ed. *The Silver Book*. Quay Books, MA Healthcare Ltd, London

Gray D, White RJ, Cooper P, Kingsley AR (2005). Understanding applied wound management. *Wounds UK* **1**(1): 62–8

Hampton S (2005) Caring for sloughy wounds. *J Community Nurs* **19**(4): 30–4

Heggers JP, Haydon S, Ko F *et al* (1992) *Pseudomonas aeruginosa* exotoxin A: its role in retardation of wound healing: the 1992 Lindberg Award. *J Burn Care Rehab* **13**(5): 512–18

Heinzelmann M, Scott M, Lam T (2002) Factors predisposing to bacterial invasion and infection. *Am J Surg* **183**: 179–90

Isenberg HD (1998) Pathogenicity and virulence: another view. *Clin Microbiol Rev* **1**(1): 40–53

Jones V (2004) Wound bed preparation and its implication for practice: an educationalist viewpoint. *Applied Wound Management Supplement 1*, Wounds UK, Aberdeen

Kingsley A (2001) A proactive approach to wound infection. *Nurs Stand* **11**(15): 50–8

Kingsley A (2003) The Wound Infection Continuum and its application to clinical practice. *Ostomy Wound Management* **49** Suppl 7A: 1–7

Kingsley A (2005) Practical use of modern honey dressings in chronic wounds. In: White R, Cooper R, Molan P, eds. *Honey: A modern wound management product*. Wounds UK, Aberdeen: 57–8

Krasner D (1995) Wound care: how to use the red-yellow-black system. *Am J Nurs* **95**(5): 44–7

Keely V (2000) Clinical features of lymphoedema. In: Twycross R, Jenns K, Todd J, eds. *Lymphoedema*. Radcliffe Medical Press, Oxford

Krasner D (1995) Wound care: how to use the red-yellow-black system. *Am J Nurs* **95**(5): 44–7

Kubo M, Van de Water L, Plantefaber LC *et al* (2001) Fibrinogen and fibrin are anti-adhesive for keratinocytes: a mechanism for fibrin eschar slough during wound repair. *J Invest Dermatol* **117**(6): 1369–81

Lamke LO, Nilsson GE, Reithner HL (1997) The evaporative water loss from burns and water permeability of grafts and artificial membranes used in the treatment of burns. *Burns* **3**: 159–65

Leaper DJ (1994) Prophylactic and therapeutic role of antibiotics in wound care. *Am J Surg* **167**(1A): 15S–20S

Lorentzen HF, Holstein P, Gottrup F (1999) Interobserver variation in the Red-Yellow-Black wound classification system. *Ugeskr Laeger* **161**(44): 6045–8

Loughry KM (1991) The III color concept for wound management. *Home Healthc Nurse* **9**(2): 28–32

Maklebust J (1997) Pressure ulcer assessment. *Clin Geriatr Med* **13**: 455–81

Meaume S, Merlin L, Guihur B (1997) Color classification of chronic wounds. A tool serving nurses. *Soins* **612**: 35–8

Moore K (2005) VAC therapy: interactions in the healing process. *Wounds UK* **1**(1): 86–93

O'Brien M (2002) Exploring methods of wound debridement. *Br J Community Nurs* **10**(12): 14

Parnham A (2002) Moist wound healing;does the theory apply to chronic wounds. *J Wound Care* **11**(4): 143–6

Rogers AA, Burnett S, Moore JC, Shakespeare PG, Chen WY (1995) Involvement of proteolytic enzymes — plasminogen activators — in the pathophysiology of pressure ulcers. *Wound Rep Regen* **3**(3): 273–3

Schein M, Wittmann DH, Wise L, Condon RE (1997) Abdominal contamination, infection and sepsis, a continuum. *Br J Surg* **84**(2): 269–72

Schultz GS, Sibbald RG, Falanga V *et al* (2003) Wound bed preparation: a systematic approach to wound management. *Wound Rep Regen* **11** (Suppl 1): S1–28

Sibbald RG, Williamson D, Orsted H, *et al* (2000) Preparing the wound — Debridement, bacterial balance, and moisture balance. *Ostomy Wound Management* **46**: 14–35

Stephens P, Wall IB, Wilson MJ *et al* (2003) Anaerobic cocci populating the deep tissues of chronic wounds impair cellular wound healing responses in vitro. *Br J Dermatol* **148**(3): 456–66

Stotts NA (1990) Seeing red and yellow and black. The three-color concept of wound care. *Nursing* **20**(2): 59–61

Tong A (1999) The identification and treatment of slough. *J Wound Care* **8**(7): 338–9

Thomas S (1997) Wound exudate — who needs it? In: Cherry G, Harding KG, eds. *Management of Wound Exudate Proceedings. Proceedings of what Joint Meeting of EWMA and ETRS Oxford 1997.* Churchill Communications, London: 1–5

Thomas S, Andrews A, Jones M (1998) The use of larval therapy in wound management. *J Wound Care* **7**: 442–52

Vowden K, Vowden P (2004) The role of exudate in the healing process: understanding exudate management. In: White RJ, ed. *Trends in Wound Care, vol III.* Quay Books, MA Healthcare Ltd, London

Vowden K, Vowden P (2003) Understanding exudate management and the role of exudate in the healing process. *Br J Nurs* **12**(20; Suppl): S4–S14

Vowden K, Vowden P (2004) The role of exudate in the healing process: understanding exudate management. In: White RJ, ed. *Trends in Wound Care, vol III*. Quay Books, MA Healthcare Ltd, London: 3–22

Villavicenzio RT (1998) The history of blue pus. *J Am Coll Surg* **187**(2): 212–16

Wall IB, Davies CE, Hill KE *et al* (2002) Potential role of anaerobic cocci in impaired human wound healing. *Wound Repair Regen* **10**(6): 346–53

Watret L (1997) Know how: management of wound exudate. *Nurs Times* **93**(30): 38–9

White RJ (2001) Managing exudate. Part 1. *Nurs Times* **97**(9): XI– XIII

White R, Cutting KF (2003) Interventions to avoid maceration of the skin and wound bed. *Br J Nurs* **12**(20): 1186–1201

Wilson JW, Schurr MJ, Le Blanc CL *et al* (2002) Mechanisms of bacterial pathogenicity. *Postgrad Med J* **78**: 216–24

Winter GD (1962) Formation of the scab and the rate of epithelialisation of superficial wounds in the skin of the young domestic pig. *Nature* **193**: 293–4

Witkowski JA, Parish LC (1982) Histopathology of the decubitus ulcer. *J Am Acad Dermatol* **6**(6): 1014–21

CASE STUDIES

Pam Cooper

Case study 1

This fifty-eight-year-old female was referred to the department of tissue viability with a pressure ulcer to her sacrum. She had been admitted to the local cancer hospice for management of her pain, following diagnosis of bowel cancer, with metastases located in her pelvis and spine. The disease process was in the terminal stages and the focus of care was pain control and comfort.

She presented with a grade 4 pressure ulcer to her sacrum (European Pressure Ulcer Advisory Panel [EPUAP], 2002). On initial examination she was in great pain, both from her underlying disease but also from her pressure ulcer, particularly at dressing changes. The wound was very malodorous, which was causing a great deal of distress both to the patient and her family.

The following treatment priorities were identified:

❖ Wound Healing Continuum: wound bed initially presented as a black/yellow wound.

Aim: to debride devitalised tissue.

Images 1–4 demonstrate an improvement in the wound bed with the debridement of the necrotic tissue. However, there still remains a yellow wound which requires further autolytic debridement.

❖ Wound Infection Continuum: there was no indication of infection present at the wound bed. However, due to the presence of devitalised tissue, the anaerobes in the wound made it very malodorous.

Aim: to treat wound as a colonised wound, but try to reduce odour.

❖ Wound Exudate Continuum: wound exudate went from medium volume/high viscosity to low volume/medium viscosity due to the breakdown of devitalised tissue.

Aim: to maintain a moist environment at the wound surface.

As the individual was in the terminal stages of her disease, the clinicians' aim was not to attempt to heal, but to improve her quality of life through symptom management. This was reflected in the dressing selection, where odour control and pain relief was of primary importance. However, the application of Applied Wound Management can still demonstrate that with palliative intervention, wounds can still move across the healing continuums. To manage her pain symptoms she was commenced on a morphine pump administered continuously through a syringe driver.

The Applied Wound Management report clearly shows a sequential improvement in the tissue present, as the wound has progressed from a black/yellow wound, to a yellow wound. The wound measurement has increased in size. This is probably due to the combined effects of wound debridement, as removing the dead tissue sees the true extent of the pressure ulcer, as well as deterioration in the individual's physical condition as the disease progresses.

This case study is a good example of how the clinician may have to alter their treatment plan to accommodate the patient's expectations, while can still progressing the wound in a positive approach.

Reference

European Pressure Ulcer Advisory Panel (2002) Guide to pressure ulcer grading. *EPUAP Review* **3**(3): 75

Case study 1

Sex: F   Date of birth: 01/02/1946

Patient notes: Bowel CA, pelvic mets, spinal mets

Wound type: pressure ulcer   Consultant: Dr Smith

Wound location: sacrum   **Referrer:** Hospital

Wound notes: No notes added

Review date: 29/08/2005 Reviewed by: Tissue viability nurse   Location: Hospice

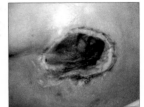

Wound continuums	**Healing:**	Black/yellow	**Wound dimensions**	**Length:**	6.5
	Infection:	Colonised		**Breadth:**	5
	Exudate:	Low/medium		**Area:**	32.5

| **Dressings used** | **Primary:** | Flamazine |
| | **Secondary:** | Allevyn |

Review notes: Conservative sharp debridement carried out to remove layer of necrotic tissue. Exposing 100% yellow adherent slough. Wound very malodorous, wound quite painful, particularly at dressing changes.

Review date: 05/09/2005 Reviewed by: Tissue viability nurse   Location: Hospice

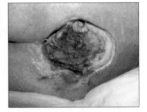

Wound continuums	**Healing:**	Black/yellow	**Wound dimensions**	**Length:**	6.5
	Infection:	Colonised		**Breadth:**	5
	Exudate:	Low/medium		**Area:**	32.5

| **Dressings used** | **Primary:** | Flamazine |
| | **Secondary:** | Allevyn Adhesive |

Review notes: Slough beginning to soften and debride particularly at wound edges. Evidence of undermining at wound edges. Odour significantly reduced.

Review date: 12/09/2005 Reviewed by: Tissue viability nurse   Location: Hospice

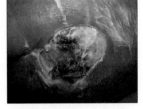

Wound continuums	**Healing:**	Black/yellow	**Wound dimensions**	**Length:**	6.5
	Infection:	Colonised		**Breadth:**	5
	Exudate:	Low/medium		**Area:**	32.5

| **Dressings used** | **Primary:** | Flamazine |
| | **Secondary:** | Allevyn Adhesive |

Review notes: No odour evident. Slough slowly debriding. 1cm undermining at wound edges. Pain reduced particularly at dressing changes.

Review date: 20/09/2005 Reviewed by: Tissue viability nurse   Location: Hospice

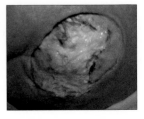

Wound continuums	**Healing:**	Black/yellow	**Wound dimensions**	**Length:**	7.5
	Infection:	Colonised		**Breadth:**	7.5
	Exudate:	Low/medium		**Area:**	56.25

| **Dressings used** | **Primary:** | Tenderwet |
| | **Secondary:** | Lyofoam Extra Adhesive |

Review notes: Wound further debrided, almost down to bone. No odour. Wound edges undermine by 1cm. Slough adherent, so treatment changed to TenderWet to facilitate debridement. Pain and odour under control.

Case study 2

A forty-four-year-old gentleman was admitted to the neurological unit following an accident on his mountain bike. He underwent anterior and posterior fixation of cervical 6 and 7. He initially made good progress and was discharged home. He was re-admitted the following day with dehiscence of his surgical neck wound, and generally unwell. He was diagnosed with meningitis and commenced on the appropriate antibiotic regime.

He was referred to the department of tissue viability for review of his wound which, on examination, measured 9cm x 4cm and 2cm in depth. On probing, the wound undermined by a further 3cm at the top following the route of the original incision.

On initial assessment, (image 1), he presented with the following:

* ❖ Wound healing continuum: a yellow/red wound, with three areas of exposed spinal vertebrae.

* ❖ Wound Infection Continuum: no infection present. Wound colonised due to its chronic nature.

* ❖ Wound Exudate continuum: exudate levels were medium volume, medium viscosity.

The clinician was initially concerned that due to the presence of exposed vertebrae and meningitis, there was no cerebral spinal fluid leak. This was ruled out and treatment commenced. The clinician was initially concerned that because of the presence of exposed vertebrae and previous treatment for meningitis, there may be cerebral spinal fluid leaking from the wound. .

Images 2 and 3 demonstrate that the wound is progressing across the continuums, with the wound bed progressing to red, there is no infection present and the exudate is reducing in volume.

The wound continues to improve with the granulation tissue coming up from the wound base and epithelialisation beginning to occur at wound edges (image 4).

Applied Wound Management clearly demonstrates the wound's natural progression from a yellow/red wound to a red/pink wound, where the wound has debrided and granulation occurs.

Case study 2

Sex: M   Date of birth: 07/05/2001

Patient notes: Neck wound following anterior and posterior fixation C6/C7. Wound dehisced following suture removal. Meningitis diagnosed and commenced on appropriate antibiotic regime.

Wound type: surgical   **Consultant:** Dr Smith
Wound location: neck   **Referrer:** Hospital

Review date: 08/08/2005 Reviewed by: Tissue viability nurse   Location: Ward A

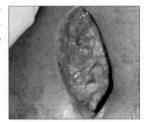

Wound continuums	**Healing:**	Yellow/red	**Wound dimensions**	**Length:**	9
	Infection:	Colonised		**Breadth:**	4
	Exudate:	Medium/medium		**Area:**	36

| **Dressings used** | **Primary:** | TenderWet |
| | **Secondary:** | Biatain Adhesive |

Review notes: Commenced on Tenderwet to facilitate wound debridement.

Review date: 12/08/2005 Reviewed by: Tissue viability nurse   Location: Ward A

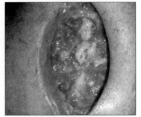

Wound continuums	**Healing:**	Yellow/red	**Wound dimensions**	**Length:**	10
	Infection:	Colonised		**Breadth:**	4.2
	Exudate:	Low/medium		**Area:**	42

| **Dressings used** | **Primary:** | Flamazine |
| | **Secondary:** | Allevyn adhesive |

Review notes: Commenced on VAC treatment regime. With black foam. Mepitel applied to the exposed spinal vertebrae to prevent any adherence to the bone.

Review date: 29/08/2005 Reviewed by: Tissue viability nurse   Location: Tissue viability out-patient clinic

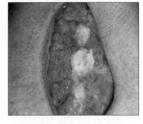

Wound continuums	**Healing:**	Red	**Wound dimensions**	**Length:**	9.5
	Infection:	Colonised		**Breadth:**	4.5
	Exudate:	Low/medium		**Area:**	42.75

| **Dressings used** | **Primary:** | Promogran Prisma |
| | **Secondary:** | Tielle |

Review notes: Lower end of wound, granulation tissue has come up to wound edge. Area of undermining at top of wound resolved. Wound depth now 1cm.

Review date: 21/09/2005 Reviewed by: Tissue viability nurse   Location: Tissue viability out-patient clinic

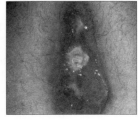

Wound continuums	**Healing:**	Red/pink	**Wound dimensions**	**Length:**	9.5
	Infection:	Colonised		**Breadth:**	4.5
	Exudate:	Low/medium		**Area:**	42.75

| **Dressings used** | **Primary:** | Promogran Prisma |
| | **Secondary:** | Allevyn Adhesive |

Review notes: Wound has very little depth to it. Area of exposed vertebrae reducing significantly.

Case study 3

Patient C was referred to our department after admission to the infection unit with an infected leg ulcer. He was twenty-seven years old and had a previous history of intravenous (IV) drug abuse. He was, however, on a treatment programme of methadone and had not been involved in drug use for some time.

He was working full-time and supporting his partner and young family. He initially knocked his ankle area while at work, causing superficial skin loss. The wound quickly presented as a locally infected painful wound.

The wound measured 8cm x 6cm and was located on his inner malleoli. It was painful at dressing changes. The ankle joint was very fixed with almost no rotational movement available.

On initial assessment (image 1), the following treatment aims were identified:

❖ Identify ulcer aetiology: a full Doppler assessment was carried out and the results identified that the ulcer was venous in nature, indicating that he would be suitable for some form of compression therapy. ABPI=1.

❖ Wound Healing Continuum: the wound bed presented as a yellow/red wound, with the slough very adherent to the wound bed. This required debridement of the yellow tissue.

❖ Wound Infection Continuum: the wound was locally infected and required active treatment with a topical antimicrobial, he was also started on IV antibiotics and then eventually stepped down onto oral antibiotics.

❖ Wound Exudate Continuum: supported the presence of infection as the wound was exuding high levels of medium viscosity exudate.

The dressing regime selected was an antimicrobial to treat the infection, covered with an absorbent hydrocapillary dressing to absorb exudate, secured with a short-stretch compression system to actively treat the leg ulcer's underlying pathophysiology. We had to change the antimicrobial regime once the exudate was reduced, as the dressing was adhering to the wound bed and causing trauma and pain on removal.

Image 2 clearly shows a reduction in wound size. The wound bed is more red than yellow, with a reduction in exudate. However, the wound remained critically colonised. As the wound improved, Patient C continued to manage his dressing changes at home and was commenced on class III compression hosiery, which he tolerated well.

The wound progressed to a red wound, but remained critically colonised, with a period of stasis (image 3). The change in the treatment regime reflects this with the clinician selecting a protease modulator to stimulate wound healing. The wound progressed to complete healing (image 4). Patient C has now been discharged from the tissue viability case load, but continues to wear his class III compression hosiery kit on both legs to prevent recurrence.

Case study 3

Sex: M   Date of birth: 03/03/1977

Patient notes: Longstanding leg ulceration due to vessel disease from IV injecting

Wound type: leg ulcer   **Consultant:** Dr Smith
Wound location: leg   **Referrer:** Hospital

Wound notes: No notes added

Review date: 27/01/2005 Reviewed by: Tissue viability nurse   Location: Tissue viability out-patient clinic

Wound continuums	**Healing:**	Yellow	**Wound dimensions**	**Length:**	8
	Infection:	Local		**Breadth:**	6
	Exudate:	High/medium		**Area:**	48

Dressings used Primary: Actisorb Silver 220
Secondary: Alione

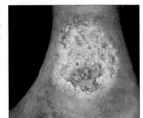

Review notes: Doppler assessment carried out. Left leg ABPI = 1.13, right leg ABPI = 1. Commenced on compression therapy using short-stretch system, setopress.

Review date: 24/03/2005 Reviewed by: Tissue viability nurse   Location: Tissue viability out-patient clinic

Wound continuums	**Healing:**	Yellow/red	**Wound dimensions**	**Length:**	4
	Infection:	Critically colonised		**Breadth:**	3
	Exudate:	Low/medium		**Area:**	12

Dressings used Primary: Acticoat
Secondary: Alione

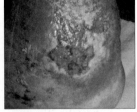

Review notes: Continued on the setopress short-stretch compression therapy.

Review date: 25/04/2005 Reviewed by: Tissue viability nurse   Location: Tissue viability out-patient clinic

Wound continuums	**Healing:**	Red	**Wound dimensions**	**Length:**	5
	Infection:	Critically colonised		**Breadth:**	3.4
	Exudate:	Medium/low		**Area:**	17

Dressings used Primary: Promogran
Secondary: Actisorb silver 220

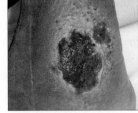

Review notes: Dressing was secured with Tielle adhesive. Continued with his class III compression hosiery, Activa 40mmHg kit.

Review date: 11/08/2005 Reviewed by: Tissue viability nurse   Location: Tissue viability out-patient clinic

Wound continuums	**Healing:**	Red/pink	**Wound dimensions**	**Length:**	0
	Infection:	Colonised		**Breadth:**	0
	Exudate:	Low/low		**Area:**	0

Dressings used Primary: Tielle Lite
Secondary: None

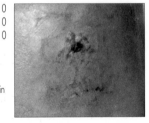

Review notes: Wound completely healed but advised Tielle while working to prevent friction and skin breakdown for a further week, but to remove once home after work. To continue to wear class III compression hosiery kit.

Case study 4

A seventy-eight-year-old lady underwent extensive bowel surgery and experienced post-operative complications, resulting in her laparotomy wound having to be re-excised three times. Unfortunately, the wound bed became necrotic, requiring further debridement and leaving no viable tissue for closure of the wound.

She presented to our department following a staff request for wound and exudate management.

On initial assessment (image 1), the wound presented with the following areas of concern:

❖ Wound Healing Continuum: the wound bed was red, however, this was due to the presence of muscle, fascia and subcutaneous tissue, with little evidence of granulation tissue.

❖ Wound Infection Continuum: clean surgical wound, which was colonised.

❖ Wound Exudate Continuum: due to the size of the wound, 22.5cm × 16.5cm, there were medium levels of low viscosity exudate exuding from the wound bed. The extent of the wound made it difficult for the staff and the patient to manage, as obtaining a seal around the wound proved difficult.

The treatment aim was to promote granulation tissue over a large surface area and prevent the complications associated with exudate management.

Images 1–5 clearly show the wound's progression, in both a reduction in the wound size and the presence of granulation tissue. The Wound Healing Continuum identifies an increase in the granulation tissue evident across the surface of the wound, progressing from a red wound to a red/pink wound, with the presence of epithelial tissue at the wounds margins. The viscosity of the exudate changes at image 5 from previously medium/low, to medium/medium, placing it in the amber zone. This may be due to the increased levels of granulation tissue, however, the clinician should be aware of this and continue to monitor, particularly for signs of infection.

The use of Applied Wound Management for this wound clearly identifies the clinician's treatment aims, but also highlights change in the wound's progress, which should be observed.

Case study 4
Sex: F   Date of birth: 01/05/1927
Wound type: surgical
Wound location: abdomen

Consultant: Dr Smith
Referrer: Hospital

Review date: 04/08/2005 Reviewed by: Tissue viability nurse   Location: Ward B

Wound continuums	**Healing:**	Red	**Wound dimensions**	**Length:** 22.5
	Infection:	Colonised		**Breadth:** 16.5
	Exudate:	Medium/low		**Area:** 371.2

| **Dressings used** | **Primary:** | TenderWet |
| | **Secondary:** | Mesorb |

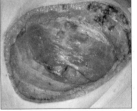

Review notes: Abdominal wound, following extensive bowel surgery requiring the laparotomy wound to be opened 3 times. Wound bed became necrotic so wound left open as no viable tissue remaining for direct closure. Wound bed shows exposed muscle and fascia, with subcutaneous tissue present at edges.

Review date: 08/08/2005 Reviewed by: Tissue viability nurse   Location: Ward B

Wound continuums	**Healing:**	Red	**Wound dimensions**	**Length:** 21.5
	Infection:	Colonised		**Breadth:** 15.5
	Exudate:	Medium/low		**Area:** 333.2

| **Dressings used** | **Primary:** | Tenderwet |
| | **Secondary:** | Mesorb |

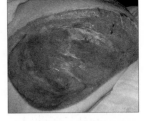

Review notes: Wound bed beginning to granulate following treatment of TenderWet. VAC treatment recommended but medical staff refused.

Review date: 24/08/2005 Reviewed by: Tissue viability nurse   Location: Ward B

Wound continuums	**Healing:**	Red	**Wound dimensions**	**Length:** 20
	Infection:	Colonised		**Breadth:** 11.5
	Exudate:	Medium/low		**Area:** 230

| **Dressings used** | **Primary:** | TenderWet |
| | **Secondary:** | Mesorb |

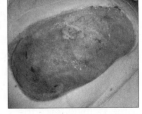

Review notes: All muscle and fascia covered by layer of granulation tissue. Wound bed red and healthy.

Review date: 08/09/2005 Reviewed by: Tissue viability nurse   Location: Ward B

Wound continuums	**Healing:**	Red/pink	**Wound dimensions**	**Length:** 17
	Infection:	Colonised		**Breadth:** 8.5
	Exudate:	Medium/low		**Area:** 144.5

| **Dressings used** | **Primary:** | Aquacel |
| | **Secondary:** | Mesorb |

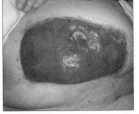

Review notes: Evidence of epithelialisation at wound edges.

Review date: 11/08/2005 Reviewed by: Tissue viability nurse   Location: Ward B

Wound continuums	**Healing:**	Red/pink	**Wound dimensions**	**Length:** 16
	Infection:	Colonised		**Breadth:** 8.5
	Exudate:	Medium/medium		**Area:** 136

| **Dressings used** | **Primary:** | Aquacel |
| | **Secondary:** | Mesorb |

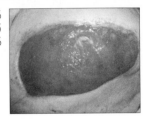

Review notes: For discharge home under the care of the district nurses.

Case study 5

A seventy-six-year-old gentleman was admitted into the intensive care unit in a collapsed unresponsive state. He presented to the department of tissue viability with a number of lower leg ulcerations, which he had been independently caring for at home with kitchen roll and toilet paper. He was septic on admission and immediately commenced on a broad spectrum antibiotic until test results confirmed where the sepsis was originating from.

On assessment (image 1), he presented with:

* Wound Healing Continuum: multiple black/yellow ulcerations to the leg which required rehydration and debridement.

* Wound Infection Continuum: *pseudomonas* infection to ulcerated areas. Odour present.

* Wound Exudate Continuum: medium volume of high viscosity exudate leaking from legs.

The treatment aim was to rehydrate and debride devitalised tissue with the use of an antimicrobial, which would reduce the presence of bacteria and reduce the levels of exudate from the wound bed.

Image 2 shows that the wound is progressing from left to right across all continuums, yellow wound, which is colonised with medium volumes of medium viscosity. This confirms to the clinician that the wound is progressing in a reasonable time-frame.

A few days later the wound is reassessed (image 3) and, although it presents with some staining from the silver antimicrobial, it continues to progress along the Wound Healing Continuum as it is now a yellow/red wound. With low volumes of high viscosity exudate, this corresponds with the autolytic debridement of the sloughy devitalised tissue.

The final review clearly demonstrates that the wounds are continuing to progress across the continuums with yellow/red, but a lot more red, healthy granulating tissue present.

The wound remains infection-free, reflected in the exudate volume.

This is a clear example of a wound's natural progression across all three continuums, reflecting the appropriate treatment interventions.

Case study 5

Sex: M   Date of birth: 04/05/1929

Patient notes: Admitted in a collapsed, confused state to the intensive care unit. He had been managing lower leg wounds at home by himself with kitchen roll and toilet paper. Poor historian due to critical condition

Wound type: leg ulcer   **Consultant:** Dr Smith
Wound location: leg   **Referrer:** Hospital

Review date: 22/04/2003 Reviewed by: Tissue viability nurse   Location: Intensive therapy unit

Wound continuums	Healing:	Black/yellow
	Infection:	Local
	Exudate:	Medium/high

Wound dimensions	Length:	6
	Breadth:	4
	Area:	24

Dressings used Primary: Flamazine
                          Secondary: Mesorb

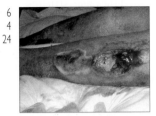

Review notes: Wound infected with *pseudomonas*. Large areas of surrounding tissue, broken and excoriated.

Review date: 29/04/2003 Reviewed by: Tissue viability nurse   Location: Intensive therapy unit

Wound continuums	Healing:	Yellow
	Infection:	Colonised
	Exudate:	Medium/high

Wound dimensions	Length:	6
	Breadth:	4
	Area:	24

Dressings used Primary: Flamazine
                          Secondary: Mesorb

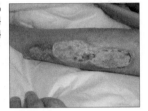

Review notes: Surrounding tissue greatly improved. Still being treated for sepsis, continued with flamazine.

Review date: 07/05/2003 Reviewed by: Tissue viability nurse   Location: Intensive therapy unit

Wound continuums	Healing:	Yellow/red
	Infection:	Colonised
	Exudate:	Low/high

Wound dimensions	Length:	6
	Breadth:	4
	Area:	24

Dressings used Primary: Granuflex (improved formulation)
                          Secondary: None

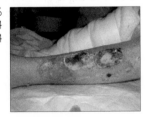

Review notes: No clinical signs of infection. All antibiotics have been stopped. Surrounding skin good. Commenced on hydrocolloid to facilitate debridement.

Review date: 23/05/2003 Reviewed by: Tissue viability nurse   Location: Intensive therapy unit

Wound continuums	Healing:	Yellow/red
	Infection:	Colonised
	Exudate:	Low/high

Wound dimensions	Length:	6
	Breadth:	4
	Area:	24

Dressings used Primary: Aquacel
                          Secondary: Allevyn

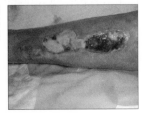

Review notes: Commenced on Aquacel as exudate levels increased due to the debridement of sloughy. Unfortunately, he passed away on 26/05/03.

Conclusion

These case studies have been designed to demonstrate both the principles of Applied Wound Management and the reports generated by AWM software.

The case studies presented offer examples of treatments selected, but may not represent all choices available.

Appendix

Applied Wound Management Tools

David Gray

Pocket guide

The pocket guide (*Figure Appendix.1*) is an A4 chart which folds into a double-sided A5 pocket guide. The front of the guide shows graphics of the three continuums, while the reverse side provides background information. The aim of this tool is to provide the practitioner with a bedside reminder of the Applied Wound Management system, and to ensure that the assessment of the patient's wound is carried out in line with the three continuums.

Figure Appendix.1: Applied Wound Management pocket guide

Assessment and documentation charts

The assessment and documentation chart comes in a two- or four-page format, and provides the practitioner with the means to collect the information recorded at each dressing change. On the front page there is space to collect basic demographic data on the patient, and baseline data relating to the wound. On the inside of the chart there are eight assessment sections. The layout of these sections allows the practitioner to compare the previous assessments and treatments at a glance (*Figure Appendix.2*). By utilising the assessment section, practitioners are encouraged to identify and document clear treatment objectives; thus promoting a systematic approach to wound management and also supporting critical evaluation of those objectives at the next consultation. At each assessment, the user is encouraged to calculate the joint score of the Wound Healing Continuum and the Wound Infection Continuum. This score is entered into a table on the front page of the chart; this is completed at each assessment allowing instant insight into the status of the wound (*Figure Appendix.3*).

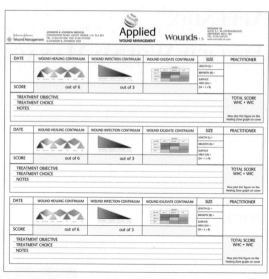

Figure Appendix.2: Assessment chart

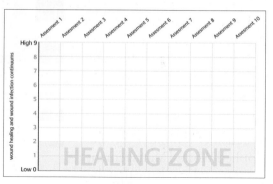

Figure Appendix.3: Assessment chart

Wall chart

The wall chart is provided in an A3 format and includes all three of the continuums. Once an assessment has been carried out at the patient's side, this chart provides the practitioner with the opportunity to identify the treatment objectives required for each continuum. For example, where black/yellow tissue has been identified, the treatment objective is to debride the necrotic/sloughy tissue (Kingsley, 2003), unless contraindicated by the patient's condition. Below the black/yellow section of the chart there is a guide to the treatment objective which states 'debride', and below this is a space where each unit/ward/team can insert its preferred option. This system not only facilitates clinical decision-making, but also promotes continuity of care among team members, as it acts as a reminder of the local protocol/formulary.

Software/database

The Applied Wound Management software has been developed with two goals in mind: to provide an easy-to-use decision support resource for practitioners; and to collate audit data about wound management practice on a much larger scale than has been done before. This benefits the individual practitioner by allowing him/her to validate his/her judgement against established standards, and benefits the wider wound care community by providing empirical data on the number and types of wounds treated, and the treatment regimes used across different clinical settings.

The software is made up of two parts: a stand-alone application that runs on the practitioner's computer, and a central data repository hosted on secure web servers, which receive anonymous audit data from the practitioners and distribute updated lists of dressings and articles for the decision-support knowledge base (see below).

❖ **Data model:** The Applied Wound Management software uses a simple data model based around patients, wounds, and reviews. Each patient can have one or more wound and each wound can have one or more reviews. The data recorded for each of these features are shown in _Table Appendix.1_. Once a patient record has been entered into the system, any number of wounds can be added for that patient without having to re-enter the patient's details. Similarly, once a wound record has been entered, any number of reviews of that wound can be incorporated.

❖ **Data entry:** The data entry forms for the application follow the data model closely. After selecting a patient from an existing list (or searching for him/her by unit number), the patient's details are shown, and the practitioner is able either to modify the patient details, or view information on the wounds recorded for that patient. Where a patient has more than one wound recorded, forward and next buttons allow practitioners to find the wound that interests them. Once the wound has been selected, the practitioner can look at the reviews of that wound, again using forward and next buttons to step through the reviews.

The user interface is split into two distinct sections: a menu section to the left of the screen; and a data-entry section to the right. The menu section is further split into two areas, with navigation items which allow the practitioner to look at a different part of the dataset (eg. to change from viewing a patient to viewing a wound, or from viewing a wound to viewing a review of that wound). Action items allow the user to make a change to the data.

With regard to entry of wound data, the menu options are context-sensitive, and change depending on what data are currently being displayed. For example, when viewing a wound record, action options are available to delete the wound record, to add a new wound record or add a new consultant; in addition, navigation options are available to return to the patient's details or to look at the reviews for the current wound, or to view a report of all the reviews of that wound.

Data are entered by selecting the appropriate value from a drop-down list. As well as making the data-entry process significantly quicker, this makes the audit process far more efficient as the same set of values is being referenced by every user of the software. To ensure that the values displayed in the drop-down lists remain current, regular updates can be transferred from the Applied Wound Management central data repository.

❖ **Wound scoring:** The process of scoring the wound during a review is instantly recognisable to anyone who is familiar with the three continuums used in Applied Wound Management. The wound is scored by clicking on the appropriate area of the graphic for each continuum, making the wound-scoring process simple and consistent.

❖ **Images:** Any images taken during a review can be added to the review record. A thumbnail picture of the default image for each review is shown on the review form at all times, and on any reports produced. The practitioner can browse the rest of the images in a gallery, and can select any of these to be the default image.

❖ **Knowledge base:** A knowledge base of reference documents is available to support the practitioner when making decisions regarding treatment. While the articles in the knowledge base can never be a substitute for clinical expertise, they provide valuable background information and details of best practice. Articles in the knowledge base are ranked according to their relevance to each of the values in each of the three continuums, allowing the practitioner to quickly find information that is appropriate to the wound he/she is treating. New or updated articles can be downloaded from the Applied Wound Management central repository as soon as they are published, ensuring that the practitioner always has access to the most up-to-date information in the field.

❖ **Reporting:** A variety of reports can be generated directly from the application. A single patient report allows a practitioner to produce a record of all the reviews that have been undertaken of the patient either since the first review, or between certain dates; in addition, a single review carried out on a specific date can be obtained. For example, if a patient attended a clinic at the end of the review, the practitioner could print off a copy of the data entered in a report format and insert it in the patient's notes. Other forms of reports relate to the workload of a particular practitioner or team.

Table Appendix.1: Data recorded

Patient	Wound	Review
Name	Wound location	Review date
Unit number	Wound type	Practitioner
Date of birth	Consultant	Review location
Sex	Referral source	Wound score
Notes	Notes	Dressings used
		Wound size
		Image(s)
		Notes

It is possible to produce reports which present the entire clinical workload of a tissue viability nurse specialist over a specified period. For example, a specialist nurse could provide a report, with or without clinical images attached, which would show each and every case that he/she has managed over a twelve-month period. This would help in providing evidence of clinical competence, and inform those not familiar with specialist practice in this area as to what can be achieved in terms of wound healing/management over a large caseload. Currently, there is limited understanding of the clinical role of the specialist practitioner in wound healing/management. Therefore, such reports would inform and educate the readers as to the variety and depth of the challenges faced on a daily basis by tissue viability nurse specialists.

Reports can be produced with all person-identifiable information removed and replaced with generic terms, allowing the reports to be distributed freely without risking a breach of the Data Protection Act.

Conclusion

Each of the tools presented above can be used individually or as part of an integrated approach to wound healing/management. The pocket guide, assessment and documentation charts, and the wall chart lend themselves to both the primary- and secondary-care settings, where teams of practitioners work together. These tools can facilitate a systematic approach to wound assessment, the identification of treatment objectives and promote continuity of care. Where an accurate Applied Wound Management assessment of the wound has been carried out, it can be documented in a quick and easy manner, allowing other practitioners to update themselves with the previous assessments and identify why a certain treatment plan was implemented. By ensuring that the local formulary or protocols appear on the wall chart, variances in treatments can be reduced and guidance provided to less expert practitioners. These three tools have the potential to facilitate high-quality care across a wide range of practice settings, by improving communication in the areas of assessment, documentation and treatment.

Applied Wound Management software has the potential to facilitate wound healing/management in both primary- and secondary-care settings, but it is on individual practice that it is likely to have an immediate impact. In relation to tissue viability specialist nurses and podiatrists, there is a tendency for their clinical role and the service that they provide not to be fully appreciated by the organisation for whom they work. By utilising the Applied Wound Management software, the practitioner can provide accurate data relating to the patients they see, generating reports for the patients' notes, and communicating effectively with other colleagues.

By producing reports which cover specific time-frames, eg. a year, and which include images, an accurate impression of the quality and impact of the service can be achieved. Such reports will leave the trust board in no doubt as to the benefits associated with specialist services in wound healing/management within the NHS. Where users of the Applied Wound Management software collaborate via the Independent Applied Wound Management Data Panel and provide anonymous data, a picture of wound healing/management in the UK can be developed. Such data will be vital in the drive to identify how many wounds are treated in the UK annually and their impact on the NHS.

Reference

Kingsley A (2003) The Wound Infection Continuum and its application to clinical practice. *Ostomy Wound Management* **49** suppl 7A: 1–7

INDEX

A

abdominal wounds 68, 87
abrasions 49
Addison's disease 20
alternating/dynamic systems 34
amputation 16, 42
anaemia 3
analgesia 44
angiogenesis 61, 68
angioplasty 9
ankle flare 38
antibiotics 43, 54
antidepressants 44
antiphospholipid syndrome 20
arterial disease 9
arteriosclerosis 9
atherosclerosis 39
atrophie blanche 6, 38
autoimmune antibodies 18
autoimmune disorders 19, 20
autolytic debridement 51, 65

B

Best Practice Statement for Compression
    Hosiery, 2005 38
biopsies 4
black wound 60
blistering 51, 53
blisters 51
burns 50
    ~ chemical burns 50
    ~ deep partial-thickness, deep dermal
        burns 51
    ~ electrical burns 50

~ full-thickness burns 52
~ radiation burns 50
~ superficial burns 51
~ superficial partial-thickness burns 51
~ thermal burns 50
burn classification 50

C

C-reactive protein (CRP) 14
cardiovascular disease 39
cavity wounds 68
celiac disease 20
cellulitis 24, 26, 74, 76
Chrohn's disease 20
chronic leg ulcers 35
claudication 7, 9
clinical audit 59, 94
complex wounds 28, 52, 54, 55
critical colonisation 84
cyanosis 37, 54
cytokines 82

D

debridement 59, 63, 64, 65, 66, 70, 76, 77,
    90, 91, 92, 93, 95, 98
debridement techniques
    clinical use of 65
decubitus ulcers 29
deep vein thrombosis (DVT) 6
dehiscence 47
dermatologists 53
diabetes 3, 7, 9, 12, 14, 15, 16, 21, 39, 41,
    42, 57
    ~ non-insulin dependent diabetes
        mellitus (NIDDM) 7

diabetic foot
  infection in 15
diabetic foot ulcers 28, 56, 79
diet 6, 9, 17, 21
Doppler 36, 37, 38, 41, 56

E

eczema 18, 21, 22, 23, 24, 26, 38

epithelialisation 68
erythema 15, 23, 24, 32, 42, 54, 58
eschar 60
excoriation 23
exudate 46, 55

F

fibrin 61, 97
fibrinogen 61
flap formation 46
free island flap 47
friction 29
frostbite 60
full-thickness skin grafts 46
fungating lesions 55
fungating tumours 52, 54
fungating wounds 54

G

gangrene 42, 60
glycosylated haemoglobin 8
gout 16, 27
grafting 46
granulation 68
Grave's disease 20
gravitational eczema 23, 24
grazes 49
growth factors 68, 73, 82
Guillan-Barré syndrome 20

H

haemo-serous fluid 51
haemostasis 81
Hashimoto's thyroiditis 20
healing 60

HEIDI 2, 3, 6, 7, 9, 10, 25
honey 64, 69, 77, 78, 89, 97
human immunodeficiency virus (HIV) 3
hydrocolloids 64, 65, 69, 78, 86
hydrogels 64, 69
hydrostatic eczema 22
hyperglycaemia 41
hyperlipaemia 39
hyperpigmentation 8
hypertension 17, 23, 37, 38, 39, 41
hypotension 54
hypothyroidism 17

I

incontinence 30
infection 1, 5, 7, 15, 18, 19, 21, 22, 24, 40,
    42, 43, 44, 45–47, 49, 51, 54, 60, 84
  spreading invasive 74
inflammatory bowel diseases 52
interdigital ulcer 12
ischaemia 29, 39, 40, 44

L

laceration 49
Lanarkshire oximetry index (LOI) 36–38
larval therapy 63
leg ulcers 28, 35, 36, 37, 38, 41, 42, 57
limb loss 42
lipodermatosclerosis 8, 38
litigation 60
lymphadenopathy 11, 24
lymphoedema 17, 74, 97
lymphoedematous limbs 80

M

maceration 62, 64, 69, 82, 95, 99
magnetic resonance imaging (MRI) 16
Marjolin's ulcer 11
matrix metalloproteinases 64
mattresses and seating 34
melanoma 60
moisture donation 69

N

necrosis 39, 44, 53, 54, 60, 61, 63, 76
necrotising fasciitis 52, 53
nephropathy 3
neuropathy 3, 12, 15, 41, 42, 43, 44, 55
non-blanching hyperaemia 32
nutrition 1, 29, 31

O

obesity 39
odour 5, 6, 7, 21, 22, 55
oral steroids 53
orthotic devices 44
osteomyelitis 3, 14, 16

P

pain 1, 5, 6, 7, 8, 9, 10, 14, 15, 16, 18, 21,
    22, 39, 42, 43, 46, 49, 51, 55, 65, 76,
    79, 82
pallor 39
patient comfort 54
pilonidal sinus excision 46
podiatrists 44, 63
polyarteritis nodosa 41
polycythaemia 17
polymyalgia rheumatica 20
positioning 33
potassium permanganate 22
pressure ulcers 28, 29, 30, 31, 33, 35, 59,
    61, 68, 82, 96, 98
Pressure Ulcer Scale for Healing (PUSH)
    33
primary closure 44–47, 49
primary dressings 87
protease enzymes 82
protease inhibitors 73
Pseudomonas aeruginosa 61, 76, 97
psoriasis 17
pus 46
pyoderma gangrenosum 52
pyrexia 54

R

radiographs 4, 14
Raynaud's phenomenon 20
reactive hyperaemia 31
rheumatoid arthritis 35, 40, 52, 55
rheumatologist 19
rotational flaps 47

S

'sausage toe' 14, 16
scleroderma 20
seating 34
secondary closure 44, 47
secondary dressings 87
secondary intention 28, 44–47, 49
septicaemia 74
serous fluid 81, 82
sharp debridement 51, 63, 65
shear 29
sickle cell disease 39
silver sulphadiazine 64
six 'Cs' 83
Sjögren's syndrome 20
skin grafts 46
skin tears 48
smoking 9
split-thickness graft 11
squamous cell carcinoma 12
squamous cell carcinoma (SCC) 11
stab wounds 49
Staphylococcus aureus 15
steri-strips 45, 49
Stirling pressure sore severity scale
    (SPSSS) 33
streptococcus pyogenes 53
stress 3
surgical debridement 54, 63
surgical excision 12
surgical wounds 28, 45, 47, 55
suturing 49
symptom control 54
systemic lupus erythematosus 41
systemic vasculitis 35, 40

T

tachycardia 54
tertiary intention 46
TIME 59, 94, 96
tissue remodelling 81
topical negative pressure therapy 68, 95
topical steroids 53
Torrance pressure sore grading scale 33
total body surface area (TBSA) 50
trauma 28, 39, 48, 49, 68
trauma wounds 28

U

urea + electrolytes 8

V

varicose veins 37
vasculitic ulcers 19, 55
vasculitis 19, 20, 26

W

Wound Bed Preparation (WBP) 59
wound bioburden 71
wound bioburden 59, 70, 71, 72, 73, 79,
    80, 81, 84, 87, 94
Wound Healing Continuum 62
wound tissue types 60

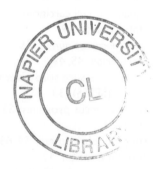